Nobody's Sleeping

Praise for *Nobody's Sleeping*

Life hacks for better sleep! Dr. John's thoughtful book provides a clear review of the anatomy, physiology, and importance of sleep. The case studies easily apply to someone we know and care about, making these lessons applicable and valuable to more than just the reader.

Through his carefully described and straightforward interventions, he provides the tools to enhance restorative sleep and gives the reader the potential to improve many aspects of physical and mental health.

A must read for those seeking to enhance the quality of their restful hours.

-Leah Cordovez, MD
Medical Director, Be Well and Flourish, Franklin, TN

Dr. John's book on sleep is an excellent resource that transcends for both patients and medical professionals. *Nobody's Sleeping* is the result of his extensive experience and knowledge in sleep medicine. The journey of his own difficulties with sleep adds a personal touch.

-Preetha Rosen, MD, DABPN, DABSM
Sleep Specialist, Gritman Sleep Center, Moscow, ID

God made our bodies to recover and sleep. Dr. Bijoy John understands the physical, spiritual, and mental need for restorative rest in a 24/7 world. Anyone who wants to sleep and stay asleep needs *Nobody's Sleeping*. It is easy to understand and practical for children, teens, and adults who need sleep. His research tells us why we need to turn off our phones at night and why we do not feel rested during the day. The "why" was most important to me to convince myself that I don't have a sleep problem. I have a schedule problem. The research alone is worth the price of the book! With anxiety and depression on the rise, this is a great resource for parents to help their families find the rhythm of restorative rest.

-Alan Clark, Lead Pastor
Gateway Community Church
GCCNaz.org / @GCCFranklin, Franklin, TN

In *Nobody's Sleeping*, Dr. Bijoy John takes us through a sweeping journey across the evolving field of sleep medicine. Through case studies, which bring to life the key aspects of how sleep affects health and well-being, and well-documented up-to-date references, we are pulled into this inspiring field.

Dr. John goes beyond traditional sleep texts to focus on important topics that are often neglected—women's health, sexual function, and athletic performance (in both adults and children). His writing style is refreshingly crisp and easy to follow and appeals to seasoned professionals as well as people outside of the medical field who want to gain a better understanding of sleep, and how we can sleep better.

Sleep is a potent healer that allows our bodies to reset and get us ready for the day ahead. My hope for readers of *Nobody's Sleeping* is that you will be inspired to sleep better, and to learn more about how we spend roughly one-third of our lives.

-Beth A. Malow, MD, MS

Burry Chair in Cognitive Childhood Development Professor of Neurology and Pediatrics, Director, Vanderbilt Sleep Division, Nashville, TN

Dr. John has written an important book on the subject of sleep and obstructive sleep apnea (OSA). As a professional in the field and someone who is passionate about the topic—having lost my sister to complications from untreated OSA—I am pleased to have found a resource that so clearly outlines the risks, symptoms, and treatment options for patients. Dr. John's writing is easy to understand and enjoyable to read. I am confident that the information provided will improve the quality and length of life for many.

-Laing Rikkers

Chairwoman and Co-Founder: Prosomnus, Inc.

Author: *Morning Leaves: Reflections on Loss, Grief, and Connection*

Just think about it for a second: we spend one-third of our lives sleeping, so have you ever wondered how to sleep well or thought about how sleep can help keep your brain and internal organs function better? Often getting the right help goes a long way.

Dr. Bijoy John has authored this wonderful book on sleep and its benefits. He covers various aspects of sleep disorders and the impact it has on various health conditions. The book also has excellent tips on how to sleep better for all age groups. I have referred several of my friends who have sleep problems to him, and they have had excellent results.

-Nepoleon Duraiswamy

Actor, Chairman, and CEO of Jeevan Technologies

Former MP and Central Minister (Government of India)

Nobody's Sleeping

7 Proven Sleep Strategies for Better Health and Happiness

Bijoy E. John, MD

NEW YORK
LONDON • NASHVILLE • MELBOURNE • VANCOUVER

Nobody's Sleeping

7 Proven Sleep Strategies for Better Health and Happiness

Published in New York, New York, by Morgan James Publishing. Morgan James is a trademark of Morgan James, LLC. www.MorganJamesPublishing.com

Proudly distributed by Publishers Group West®

ISBN 9781636983554 paperback
ISBN 9781636983561 ebook
Library of Congress Control Number: 2023948285

Cover Design by:
Rachel Lopez
www.r2cdesign.com

Interior Design by:
Christopher Kirk
www.GFSstudio.com

To my patients
You have taught me to be a better physician

Download Your FREE Special Report

The Good, the Bad, the Ugly... and the Beautiful

How a Continuous Positive Airway Pressure (CPAP) Machine Can Help You Sleep Better, Feel Sexier, and Live Longer

Are you or your partner tired of restless nights, daytime exhaustion, and disruptive snoring that makes life miserable… but hesitant to get (or use) a CPAP because of all the "issues"?

You're not alone! In my FREE special report, you'll learn how CPAP therapy can:

- Give you (and your partner) "the gift of bliss"—peaceful, uninterrupted sleep
- Restore your vitality, cognitive function, and memory
- Help you wake up feeling refreshed and energized
- Boost your mood and overall well-being throughout the day

You'll also discover…

- How to make nighttime CPAP preparation as simple as brushing your teeth
- How to reduce the adjustment period when first using your CPAP
- 5 ways to overcome CPAP "stigma"
- 10 top reasons why people abandon using their CPAP (a huge health risk!)
- How to prevent problems like "rainout" or "dry throat" before they begin
- How to clean your CPAP—and avoid the one *most dangerous* thing you can do when using a CPAP (besides not using it!)
- How to *enhance* intimacy with your partner by using a CPAP
- How to get your partner to actually *want* to use a CPAP every night without fail

Don't let one more sleepless night affect your health, your confidence, or your relationship. Using a CPAP could be your ticket to a sleeping better, feeling sexier, and living longer! To claim your FREE special report, visit SleepFixAcademy.com/CPAP or simply scan the QR code below.

Disclaimer

The information provided in this book is intended for general informational purposes only and should not be considered as a substitute for professional medical advice, diagnosis, or treatment. Always seek the advice of your physician or other qualified health providers with any questions you may have regarding a medical condition.

The author does endorse select treatments and products mentioned in this book.

Any resemblance of characters portrayed in this book to real individuals, living or deceased, is purely coincidental and unintentional. The people, events, and situations depicted in this book are a product of the author's imagination and creativity. While some people may possess certain traits, behaviors, or attributes that might resemble those of real people, any similarities are not meant to imply direct connections or representations of actual individuals.

Table of Contents

Acknowledgments

Writing a book has been harder than I imagined and writing it while running a medical practice has been challenging. I could not have done it without the love and support of many wonderful people.

This book would not have happened without my wife, Dotty. She has always believed in me, and she was the first one to notice that I had a powerful message. She has been my inspiration to write this book, and it would not have gone anywhere without her love and constant encouragement.

I am indebted to my children Brandon and Rachael for their constructive criticisms and being the guinea pigs on whom I was able to experiment my treatment plans.

I want to thank my good friend and fellow author Ray Mullican who was the first one whom I had approached with the idea of writing a book, and he was helpful in guiding me through this process.

I also want to thank my colleagues and friends Drs. Bitten Young, Preetha Sharone, Beth Malow, Meenakshi Prabhakar, Leah Cordovez, Sri Moturi, Murugusundaram, and Stephen May for taking the time out of their busy schedules and helping with editing and being a constant source of encouragement.

I want to thank Derek Schraw, Pastor Mark Karls, and Marilynn Halas for grammatical edits and for helping to keep the content relevant.

I am always grateful to visionary Aaron Stokes for getting this whole process started and bringing out the entrepreneur in me.

I want to thank Laura DeAngelis for helping with all the illustrations.

Many thanks to fellow author Traci Barrett for being always available and helping me with the finer points in this production.

There are not enough words to appreciate Alice Sullivan who was instrumental in adding friendly content and making my book readable for everyone. She was on cue all the time and was very prompt and was able to keep up with me every step of the way. I plan to collaborate with her for my next book.

Writing a book is a team effort, and Adéle Booysen greatly contributed her editorial skills to make this book the best that it can be. I also want to thank my publisher, Morgan James Publishing, for their belief in me and the message of this book.

Of course, I could not have done it without Karen Anderson, my strategic book coach and associate publisher with Morgan James Publishing, who has her unique style of challenging me. Her guidance and editing were most crucial in delivering the content and I could not have done this without her. It has been a long and arduous process, but I have enjoyed it thoroughly and I cannot wait to write several books with her help.

I am eternally grateful to my late mom, Mrs. Annamma John, for her many sacrifices and inspiring me to do the very best in everything I do. I am sure she is smiling from above enjoying this accomplishment.

I want to thank my dad, P. O. John, for lifting me up when I thought it was impossible. His gentle encouragement has helped to make this happen.

I also want to thank my family members and friends who have constantly supported me in this endeavor and my colleagues who have placed their trust in me by referring their patients and family members into my care.

Many others have been inspirational and helpful in this endeavor, and if I have failed to mention it is purely unintentional.

I have made every effort to make the content relevant and accurate. If there are any errors or omissions, I take full responsibility.

Finally, I am deeply thankful for the Almighty for helping me with this effort for he is the provider of Ultimate Sleep.

Foreword

You may wonder why a cardiologist is writing the foreword to a book about sleep disorders. The answer is simple. A large proportion of the patients I treat in my cardiology practice either suffer from poor sleep or have sleep disorders, and getting good quality sleep is an essential component of optimal cardiac health. I often refer my patients to sleep specialists.

Over my years in practice, I have been fortunate to call Dr. Bijoy John, the author of this book, a highly valued colleague and friend. He has dedicated his professional life to the thoughtful diagnosis and treatment of sleep disorders. He knows all too well that most people find good quality sleep elusive, and that many do not have easy access to a sleep specialist. Dr. John has written this book to teach all of us what healthy sleep is, how to attain it, and why you really ought to care.

The most common sleep disorder in my cardiac patients is sleep apnea. Sleep apnea is not a minor problem that can be safely ignored. Far from an innocent bystander, it is a driver of many heart-related conditions. These include high blood pressure, atrial fibrillation, heart attack, stroke, heart failure, and serious heart rhythm problems. It can make heart disease difficult or impossible to treat. Untreated sleep apnea can even lead to sudden death.

I am a strong proponent of identifying and treating sleep apnea in particular, because doing so improves heart health and in many cases treating it can save lives. It is also worth noting that appropriate treatment is often life-changing for the patient. Not infrequently, a patient who begrudgingly agreed to a consultation with Dr. John will return to my office a year later and say, "Doc, I just have to thank you. Getting my sleep apnea treated has absolutely changed my life for the better. I would never have believed it. I feel great. My blood pressure is better. Even my cholesterol is better. I've lost a few pounds. I wake up with energy and I have even started to exercise! I feel better than I have in 20 years!"

That said, this book is not just for cardiac patients with sleep apnea. That is only one of many topics covered within it. It is for everyone—from small children to great-grandparents, from athletes to executives, from college students to entire families.

You may assume that your cardiologist or primary care physician has already considered whether you might have sleep apnea or another sleep disorder. You may believe he or she would have already referred you to see a sleep specialist if you needed it. However, to be frank, your cardiologist is probably not thinking about sleep disorders in the very limited time he or she has been allotted to see you at your annual appointment. If sleep disorders are even on their list, they fall well below the more widely recognized (though not more important) cardiovascular risk factors: control of cholesterol, hypertension, diabetes, weight, smoking, physical inactivity. The same likely goes for your primary care physician.

Therefore, recognizing sleep problems starts with you. This book provides a road map to sleep success, with actionable insights and clear instructions on when expert consultation is required. It has all the information you need to learn what healthy sleep ought to be.

Even if you do not have a sleep disorder, it is likely that your sleep could be improved. You will learn many effective techniques that can be implemented at home to improve the quality of your sleep, and the sleep of your entire family.

What you learn as you read may even save your life, or the life of a loved one. This book serves as an invaluable resource in your journey toward optimal health.

-Britten F. Young, MD

Cardiologist, Nashville, TN

A Note from the Author: Why I Care

It was 4:06 a.m.

I awoke to my pager beeping and vibrating across the bedside table. I winced. I had already been awake for almost 24 hours during this on-call shift at the hospital, and getting jerked out of my first catnap in a full day was painful.

I sat up, rubbing my eyes and trying to shake the last lingering impressions of a dream. The pager alarm meant that a patient was coding (having a cardiac arrest). So, as much as gravity and exhaustion were pulling me back to bed, I needed to get moving. . . and get moving *fast*.

As I stepped out of my on-call room into the fluorescent hallways of the hospital and started to run toward the code, I told myself I needed to dig deep and rally all my remaining energy and focus—a person's life was at grave risk.

When I reached the patient's room, I surveyed the person and the monitors around the room. The machines were dinging and chirping, alerting us to the patient's dropping oxygen levels and other troubling vital signs. Immediately, adrenaline took over, and I started giving instructions to the nurses and respiratory therapists.

Thank goodness the patient survived.

But even as I performed my essential duty—telling the staff when to perform CPR, when to administer drugs, when to pull out the defibrillator—I was realizing in the back of my mind that my current sleep schedule was completely unsustainable. There was no way I could always be at my best on such a scant amount of sleep.

There was *no way* anyone could.

Med school and fellowship training required me to stay up late or pull all-nighters (they are working on changing this for young doctors), but I knew the immense impact it had on me the next day. It felt overwhelming.

Fortunately, medical residencies and fellowship training don't last forever, and I was able to recover a healthy sleep rhythm once I completed my training. My normal sleep habits once again coincided with the natural circadian rhythms of my body, not the hospital's frenetic schedule.

But what I learned about the negative consequences of sleep deprivation stuck with me. I'll never forget the way lack of sleep clouded my concentration or the fatigue that followed me around like a shadow, even while I was tasked with the all-important business of saving lives.

As a pulmonary and critical care doctor, although I saved hundreds of lives working in the intensive care unit (ICU), it soon became clear to me I was using "reactionary medicine." I was treating things *after* the fact and, in some cases, it was sadly too late.

I also began noticing that most of my patients—whether they were in the hospital or not—weren't getting the deep, restorative sleep that they desperately needed. Even more concerning, the lack of sleep was harming their bodies in profound ways. People who were sleep-deprived were more likely to suffer from high blood pressure, uncontrolled blood sugar, poor memory and cognition, and even premature death. Their organs simply didn't function as well as the people who were getting an adequate amount of restful sleep.

Poor sleep also meant they were more likely to make mathematical and judgment errors, report poor work performance, and struggle with mental illness. This was more profound in the hospital setting, especially in the ICU, where people could hardly sleep, which resulted in patients being delirious.

When I was an attending physician in the ICU, there was one patient in particular who provided the lightbulb moment that changed my focus and my life's work.

I got paged and was called in to see Andre, a 58-year-old male who was admitted to the ICU with acute onset stroke with complete paralysis of his right side. His blood pressure was 220 over 110, and he was hardly breathing. I placed him on a respirator (breathing machine) immediately to keep him alive.

His lab work showed he had uncontrolled diabetes. The electrocardiogram showed he had atrial fibrillation, an irregular heart rhythm. Andre's wife of 30 years,

Mandy, was sitting in the chair next to his bed crying hysterically, fearing she might lose him. (Remarkably, Andre had the stroke while he was visiting his friend in the hospital. It would have been highly unlikely he would have survived if he had been anywhere else.)

Days turned into weeks, and Andre finally turned the corner. He ended up spending three weeks in the ICU and then he did four months of physical therapy to regain his strength. He still has partial weakness on his right side, and he uses a cane to get around.

While he was in the hospital, I ordered several tests, including a sleep study, which showed he had *severe* sleep apnea. We immediately started him on CPAP (continuous positive airway pressure) therapy.

Mandy informed me Andre's blood pressure had been high for the past year, and his doctors had tried several medications to control this. She also admitted he was snoring loudly at night and had pauses in his breathing. Mandy along with Andre's family doctor had been insisting that he see a sleep specialist, but he didn't like the idea of sleeping in a strange place to get a sleep study, and he had a variety of other excuses since he thought he was "just fine."

Sadly, after his stroke, he wasn't "just fine" anymore. For me, it was clear that the one unifying cause of his uncontrolled blood pressure, diabetes, and heart rhythm was his *untreated sleep apnea*. It hit me like a ton of bricks that if his sleeping issues had been identified and treated earlier, it's unlikely he would have been at risk for his life.

That's when I decided I wanted to be proactive and help my patients avoid these serious conditions *before* they started. And I believed that making sure they got the deep sleep that they needed would make a significant improvement in their quality of life.

I knew then, and I know now, good sleep is essential.

My Journey to Becoming a Doctor

Although I've lived in the USA for more than 30 years now, I was born into a hard-working, middle-class family in Chennai, a city on the southeast coast of India, the youngest of three children to my parents, P. O. John and Annamma John.

Ours was a typical Indian family. My dad was the sole breadwinner and worked for the government, and my mom was a schoolteacher and a homemaker who dedicated her life to taking care of her children.

But when I was just a baby, an event happened that changed the whole trajectory of our family.

I was 11 months old when my mom and I were involved in a terrible bus accident in which several people were killed.

I was sitting on my mom's lap when the bus rolled over, and when it was all over, I was found still clinging to her as she protected me. I somehow escaped relatively unharmed, but my mom suffered third-degree burns on her legs. She spent close to a year in the hospital.

Because my father had to work full time, our young family was divided up until my mother was released from the hospital. During that year, I lived with my maternal grandfather (my mom had lost her mother at a young age), my sister stayed with my father, and my brother lived with our paternal grandparents.

My mom always loved children and she loved teaching, but after the accident, she had to give up teaching as she could no longer walk. Still, she believed with all her heart that a good education was the key to success. So, when we were reunited as a family, my mother provided everything we needed to excel academically. Study, we did!

All three of us became the valedictorian of our classes. My brother went on to pursue engineering, my sister became a teacher like our mom, and I became a doctor.

My interest in medicine was rooted in my childhood experiences with severe asthma. I loved sports, but I couldn't play like the other kids, as playing sports resulted in shortness of breath—a scary experience, to say the least.

I was very close to my mom, and when my mom faced a decision whether to amputate her legs due to the severity of her injuries, there was one doctor who stood strong and assured her he would do everything he could to save her legs. . . and he did.

The exceptional care that was shown to my mom and me when I was young molded me into the person and physician that I have become—the type of doctor who made a difference. I am honored to have been able to help many people in life-and-death situations throughout my career.

But healing has more elements than just the physical. Born into a Syrian Orthodox Christian family, faith still plays a huge part in my life. For me, one of the greatest testimonies of the role faith plays in healing was watching my mother's profound faith in her journey to recovery.

The Syrian Orthodox Church in India comes from the first church started by the disciples in AD 52, after Christ's death. The legend goes that "doubting Thomas" preached Christianity in the area I was born. Thomas had converted lots of Hindus in that region of which the descendants still adhere to their faith. I would even study at St. Thomas Mount, built on the hill where Thomas was persecuted and killed.

Upon completing my undergraduate studies in India, my passion to excel and provide exceptional service landed me in the USA to pursue my higher education. That is where I discovered for the first time what had caused my asthma issues. I found it so fascinating to know how our lungs work, and I decided to specialize in pulmonary medicine. And since many people land in the ICU when they are having difficulty breathing, I also trained in intensive care medicine.

It was during my pulmonary/critical care fellowship training at the University of Tennessee (Memphis) in the late nineties that one of my professors who knew my interest in trying to help people in the ICU sleep better (we know we heal when we sleep) urged me to explore the field of sleep medicine. So, I turned my focus to the underserved field of sleep medicine and also completed a fellowship in sleep medicine.

It had always seemed to me that it wasn't rocket science to understand that there was a huge correlation among the study of breathing, the study of sleeping, healing, and quality of life. I was actually surprised that medical students didn't spend more time studying about sleeping in med school.

Thinking back, I have always loved to sleep, and I think I intuitively knew how vital sleep was. My mom instilled good sleep habits at home—she was a big fan of afternoon naps. She made sure everyone in the household took a nap. (I enjoy a good nap even to this day. My family knows if it's 2:30 on a Sunday afternoon and they can't find me—I'm napping!)

But even though I have studied sleeping all my life, like many people, I too, have struggled with insomnia.

After my dear mom passed away in 2014, the daily grief I felt was terrible and I often struggled with insomnia. My sadness would often penetrate my sleep and I longed for a deeper rest.

When I left the hospital environment to go into private practice, I would often wrestle with overwhelming thoughts at night—like many business owners do.

And as a middle-aged man, I too, found myself vulnerable to sleep apnea as my wife, Dotty, can attest! (I did a home sleep study and consulted with a fellow sleep doc since I was the patient.) I've been using a CPAP for a year now with great results. There are also exciting new technologies coming on the market—I am now trying out a new device eXciteOSA®, a daytime treatment for sleep apnea.

Now, after many years of study and personal experience, I have identified *7 Proven Sleep Strategies* to help you sleep better, be more productive, and live happier.

The strategies and techniques that my patients and I have used over the years work. They sleep well and I sleep well.

As I look back on my life, I realize my experience with asthma and struggling to breathe made me a better pulmonologist. I also realize that the same is true with insomnia and sleep apnea—I know what it's like to struggle with sleep.

For decades now, it has been my life's goal to help others wake up in the morning refreshed and rejuvenated after a restful night of sleep.

When one of my patients asks, "Do you know how awful it feels not to sleep and can I really get better?"

I can say with certainty, "Yes, I do know, and yes, there's definitely hope."

Chapter 1

Warning Signs You May Have Sleep Issues

Does any of this sound familiar?

When someone asks you how you are, you often reply, "I'm tired."

Your family says you're cranky all the time.

Your spouse is constantly pushing and kicking you during the night because of your snoring, so you're irritated with them, and they're irritated with you.

You're not doing well at work, and everyone is annoying you.

You oversleep often (or hit the snooze button multiple times) or fall asleep at work.

Your medication isn't helping your blood pressure or your diabetes, even though you take it consistently.

Your libido is waning or nonexistent (and you're not that old!)

You wake up in the middle of the night, grab your phone, and then can't go back to sleep.

You find yourself prowling the kitchen and grabbing a snack at 3 a.m.

You stay up way too late on your phone scrolling social media or checking email.

You set your alarm for 6 a.m. but you find you're waking up at 3 a.m. and can't go back to sleep.

You always worry about falling asleep because you hate that "draggy" feeling when you wake up.

You sometimes feel like you've got the flu because you're just *sooo* tired.
You find yourself not remembering things or making "stupid" careless errors.
You've tried every over-the-counter sleep aid (even cannabis) to help you go to sleep at night.
Your evening glass of wine has become two to four glasses just to help you relax and fall asleep.
You eat (or overeat) just because you're tired and don't have the energy to say no, and sweets or carbs make you feel better.
You're tired of being tired.

The "Not so Obvious" Impact of Sleep Issues

Sadly, sleep disorders are slow killers.

There is no pain or immediate cause and effect. Bad sleep habits are often *years* in the making. We all can pick up bad habits from a young age and this becomes the norm. When we're young, it is easier to cope with sleep debt from days or even months of not sleeping well.

But as time goes on, there are more responsibilities—like having a stressful job, meeting deadlines, raising a family, facing medical and emotional illnesses, loss, bereavement, not to mention the time changes that happen every spring and winter.

It is easy to take a pill or try a new hack that you found on the internet. But the road to good sleep is like taking the stairs; there are no quick fixes. It's about discipline and creating sleep-positive routines and staying clear of all the misinformation.

But as we all know, sleep is *absolutely essential* to all aspects of life.

We need sleep for learning, eating well, performing athletically, having sex, feeling well emotionally, and maintaining healthy relationships. So, if sleep is so important, why are so few people getting help for their sleep disorders?

Most people wrongly assume that sleep is far less important than it is. Even though they may be suffering from poor sleep for several reasons, they don't consider it to be bad enough to seek help. For many who are interested in seeking help, they worry that there will be a delay in getting to see a sleep physician and that the testing will be cumbersome, expensive, or uncomfortable.

Also, people assume that the diagnostic process for a sleep disorder like apnea is arduous and requires staying overnight in a strange place with several wires hanging off their body while also being monitored on camera.

Thankfully, home testing has revolutionized the field of sleep diagnostic methodology and there is no need to go to a strange place for testing. Apart from rare instances where a person would need to be monitored in-person overnight, you can have your sleep assessed in the comfort of your own home. Furthermore, home testing is more accurate than ever, and comparable to an in-lab study.

But the main reason why people don't seek help early is the fact that sleep problems can seem trivial, even though they're quite serious. Sleep problems don't "hurt", and you don't notice disrupted sleep and snoring when you are asleep.

My goal (and hope) is for you and your whole family to sleep better.

The process of going to sleep is an art. It takes time, patience, and discipline. At times, you may fall off the band wagon due to life events, but by following the *7 Proven Sleep Strategies*, you can get back on it.

I tend to think of the mind like a revved-up jet engine. Just like a pilot must prepare for landing and bringing the plane to a stop, you should do the same for easing in to sleep.

Getting to sleep is not an on–off switch (though we all wish it were), but rather a dimmer, and there is no way around that. That's why it's important to not consume stimulants, like caffeine, or doing things to accelerate your mind, like being on the phone or listening to loud music prior to sleep if we want to sleep well.

Thankfully, if you are struggling to sleep well, you don't have to wait till the effects are irreversible. It's easier than ever to get help with your conditions.

I have outlined all the necessary guidelines to empower you to gain control of your sleep. I have also included the Sleep Journal and Sleep Assessment available at the back of this book, or you can download printable versions at SleepFixAcademy.com. Using these will help you to identify potential pitfalls and sleep-negative routines you may have picked up over time.

With advances in the diagnostic methodology, getting better sleep should be a seamless and even pleasant experience for people. There are better treatment options and innovative medications to treat various sleep disorders.

Getting treatment now rather than later means that you'll feel better, sooner. Plus, you'll reduce your risk for a host of different health issues, meaning that you'll likely live a longer, more productive, and healthier life.

Even better, most health insurance now covers testing and treatment for sleep issues. You can get the help you need with less hassle and less money out of pocket than ever before.

Here Are Some Indicators That You May Have Sleep Issues

Daytime sleepiness: Feeling excessively tired and sleepy during the day, even after supposedly getting a full night's sleep, can indicate insufficient sleep or other sleep disorders.

Fatigue, low libido, and low energy levels: If you constantly feel drained, lack energy, and struggle to stay focused and alert throughout the day, it could be a sign of sleep deprivation.

Poor concentration and memory problems: Sleep deprivation can impair cognitive function, leading to difficulties with concentration, memory recall, and overall mental performance.

Snoring and sleep pauses: Snoring and stopping breathing at night are signs of sleep apnea.

Rapid movements in sleep: Sudden movements like kicking and punching or kicking your legs could be signs of sleep disorders like REM behavior disorder (RBD) or periodic limb movement disorder (PLMD).

Mood swings and irritability: Lack of sleep can make you more irritable, short-tempered, and prone to mood swings. You may find it challenging to regulate your emotions effectively.

Increased appetite and cravings: Sleep deprivation can disrupt the hormones that regulate hunger and appetite, leading to increased cravings for unhealthy foods and potential weight gain.

Reduced immune function: Chronic sleep deprivation weakens the immune system, making you more susceptible to illnesses and infections.

Impaired physical coordination: Insufficient sleep can affect motor skills, balance, and coordination, increasing the risk of accidents and injuries.

Reduced productivity and performance: Lack of sleep can negatively impact your ability to concentrate, solve problems, and make decisions, resulting in decreased productivity at work or school or in sports.

Frequent headaches: Sleep deprivation can trigger headaches and migraines in some individuals.

Microsleep episodes: Brief episodes of involuntary sleep, known as microsleep, can occur when you are sleep-deprived. These episodes may last only a few seconds but can be dangerous, especially if they happen while driving or operating machinery.

If you consistently experience one or more of these warning signs, it's important to prioritize getting adequate sleep by adopting the *7 Proven Sleep Strategies*, and if necessary, consulting a healthcare professional for further guidance.

Chapter 2

Desperate for Sleep

Michael Jackson, the King of Pop, was an iconic American singer, songwriter, and dancer. Jackson revolutionized the music industry with his unique blend of pop, rock, and soul and became one of the most influential and best-selling artists of all time.

But Michael had a problem that, ultimately, sucked him into a deep hole of darkness.

Throughout his life, Michael struggled with debilitating sleep issues. The demands of his career, constant touring, and the pressures of fame often led to high levels of stress and anxiety which, along with his workaholic nature and perfectionism, exacerbated his sleep problems.

He was known to work late into the night, which disrupted his sleep/wake cycle and further contributed to his sleep troubles, deeply affecting both his physical and mental well-being. He was often getting only four hours of sleep or less per night.

To cope with his unbearable insomnia, Michael sought various treatments and remedies to provide the relief he so desperately desired. The singer was known to try everything from vitamin treatments to prescription medications to help him sleep; however, over time, they became increasingly ineffective.

Michael's physical and mental well-being began to deteriorate. He was chronically sleep-deprived, and it took a significant toll on his energy levels, cognitive function, and emotional stability.

He spiraled deeper and deeper in his desperation to sleep and ultimately turned to propofol, a potent intravenous sedative-hypnotic medication used primarily for anesthesia during surgical procedures. (The drug works by enhancing the activity of the neurotransmitter GABA—a gamma-aminobutyric acid—in the brain, which leads to sedation, relaxation, and loss of consciousness.)

Tragically, Jackson died in 2009. His official cause of death, as determined by the Los Angeles County Coroner's Office, was acute propofol and benzodiazepine intoxication.

The combination of these medications led to profound respiratory depression, which resulted in cardiac arrest and caused his death.

Ultimately, Michael Jackson died from lack of sleep.

He was 50 years old.

Why Do We Need to Sleep?

Most of us would agree that sleep is essential for children. We know that their little bodies are growing, and sleep is an undisputed part of their health and growth process. (If you've ever been around a cranky toddler or teenager, it can be pretty obvious when they're overtired!)

But good sleep isn't just necessary for children. In fact, adequate sleep is essential at every age, for a host of different functions beyond simply recharging.

Sleep is when our bodies consolidate memories, strengthen our immune systems, repair our muscles, regulate our hormones, resolve psychological conflicts, and more. Sleep also gives our essential organs a chance to take a rest. The functioning of various organs—notably the heart, lungs, and brain—is drastically reduced to conserve energy and get ready for optimal functioning the next day. And human growth hormone in children is maximally secreted in deep sleep, and sound sleep is needed for their optimal growth.

When we're asleep, we are free to dream and run our imagination wild, resolve problems and wake up refreshed. Oh, how we crave that feeling of waking up energized and ready to tackle the day!

Despite how critical sleep is, a recent survey found many of us (I'd venture to say *most* of us) aren't getting enough. A study evaluating sleep in adults reported that most adults feel sleepy about three days a week, with many reporting it affects their daily activities, mood, mental acuity, and productivity.[1]

More than 60 million adults suffer from poor sleep quality or sleep disorders, like sleep apnea and insomnia.[2] And 70% of children, including many teenagers, also struggle with one or more sleep issues per week.[3]

When you don't get enough sleep, many fundamental processes are compromised. Sleep deprivation affects thinking, concentration, energy levels, and mood.

In fact, sleep is "essential for optimal physical health, immune function, mental health, and cognition," reports the National Institutes of Health.

The way you feel while you're awake depends in part on what happens while you're sleeping. During sleep, your body is working to support healthy brain function and maintain your physical health. The damage from sleep deficiency can occur in an instant (such as a car crash), or it can harm you over time. For example, ongoing sleep deficiency can raise your risk for some chronic health problems like high blood pressure and diabetes. It also can affect how well you think, react, work, learn, and get along with others."[4]

Individuals with insomnia generally have adequate time and opportunity to sleep but have difficulty falling asleep, even though they feel fatigued during the day. They may also have difficulty maintaining sleep or returning to sleep after waking up. Insomnia is reportedly one of the most common medical complaints, generating more than five million medical office visits each year in the United States.

People with insomnia are usually unhappy with the quality of their lives and report increased fatigue, sleepiness, confusion, tension, anxiety, and depression.

So, if sleep is such an essential natural process, why is it so hard to come by for so many people?

The truth is, no matter what phase of life you're in, sleep is an incredibly complex (and still somewhat mysterious) process.

Changes in Sleep Patterns During the Night

Sometimes, when talking about sleep and sleep disorders, it's helpful to know some of the science behind why we sleep.

During a normal sleep period, we all progress through four to five sleep cycles, and each of those cycles is made up of sleep stages. These stages of sleep are then broken down into two categories: rapid eye movement (REM) and non-REM sleep.

Understanding the distinction between the two categories is important because what happens during REM sleep is dramatically different from what happens during the non-REM stages.

Within REM there are two phases (tonic and phasic), and in non-REM there are three stages (stages 1, 2, and 3).

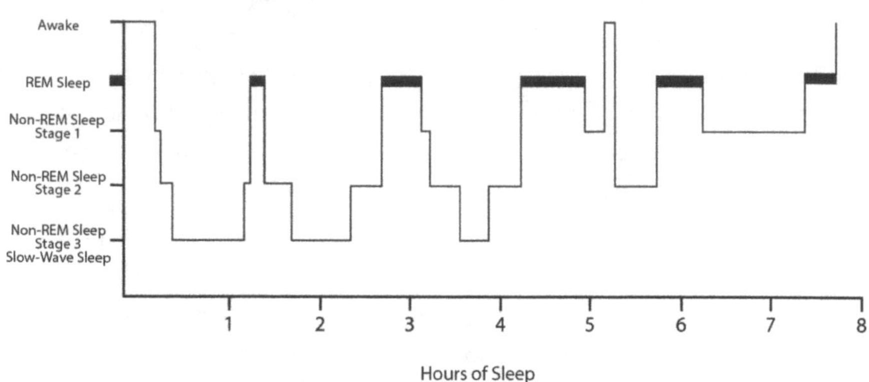

FIGURE 1. Sleep Stages

We enter the sleep state through non-REM sleep in stage 1. This stage is short, representing the act of dozing off and transitioning into sleep. In stage 2, the body and mind slow down as you settle into sleep. It's easiest to be awoken during these first two stages.[5]

Next, we progress to stage 3, also known as deep sleep or slow-wave sleep, where the body is in recovery mode, slowing down even further. Overall brain activity slows, a telltale pattern of reduced activity; this is considered deep and restful sleep.

From there, we enter REM sleep. During REM periods, the body is still, but our brain remains quite active. A brain in REM sleep resembles a brain that's fully awake, partly because REM sleep is when we experience most of our dreams. Breathing and heart rate are erratic during REM cycles, but most of the muscles—except our eye muscles and the diaphragm (which we need for breathing)—are paralyzed.

Though REM is not restful, it's instrumental in mental and emotional healing. It is the sleep stage in which internal conflict resolution occurs. (More dreams happen in REM sleep.) Many psychiatric conditions, especially depression, are correlated with some alterations in the REM sleep pattern.

Each sleep cycle takes between 60 and 120 minutes. And in the early part of the night, more time is spent in non-REM sleep. REM sleep normally occurs roughly around 90 minutes into sleep and is denser later in the night, especially from 2–5 a.m.) (See Figure 1.)

Each stage has a unique wavelength and frequency, which is measured by EEG (electroencephalogram) electrodes placed on the scalp. When you are awake, the frequency is fast. Once your eyes are closed and you begin to fall asleep, the waves slow down. The waves are slowest in stage 3 sleep (deep sleep) and appear more chaotic in REM sleep.

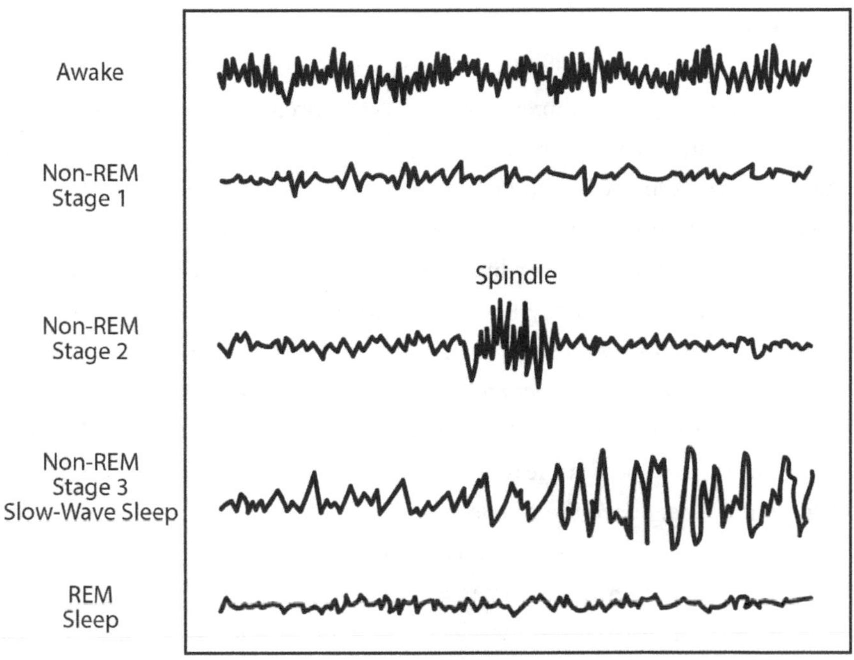

FIGURE 2. EEG of Brain Waves During Sleep
During Non-REM Stage 1 sleep, the frequency of brain waves is slightly slower than when awake. During Non-REM Stage 2 sleep, the frequency is slower with short occasional burst of rapid frequencies called sleep spindles. During Non-REM Stage 3 sleep, the frequency is much slower. In REM sleep, the brain waves are chaotic and have a sawtooth appearance.

External and Internal Sleep Cues

Our bodies take cues to sleep from two different sources: our internal sleep drive and our external indicators. The internal sleep drive is also referred to as homeostatic pressure—as this pressure builds up, so does your desire for sleep. It's low in the morning, and the pressure accumulates as the day goes by.

Beyond the internal drive, our bodies also take their sleep cues from the environment; this is called *circadian alert signaling*. This simply means that our bodies follow the rhythm of daytime and nighttime. When we're in sync with the outside world, we naturally wake up when the sun rises, and we get sleepy when the sun goes down. This is part of the reason people living in extreme northern areas, like Alaska or Norway, where the days and nights can last a full 24 hours, often struggle to regulate their sleep.

A part of the brain called the suprachiasmatic nucleus (pronounced *su·pra·chi·as·mat·ic* nucleus, abbreviated as SCN), located in the hypothalamus, helps to regulate our circadian rhythms and helps our body stay attuned to these environmental influences. Our SCN also makes us drowsy at certain periods of the day.

During the afternoons, typically from 1:30 p.m. to 3:30 p.m., and early mornings, from 2 a.m. to 4 a.m., our bodies enter a natural lull when we start to feel drowsy. This is the natural body rhythm due to the dimming of the SCN. During these times, we are more vulnerable to mistakes, errors, and accidents.

Have you ever gone to a meeting at 2 p.m.? Most everyone is aware that they are not at the top of their game, and the meetings are typically not as productive as early morning meetings. It stands to reason that meetings at this time should be rare if you want to get the most out of the people attending.

Some high-level executives will even sneak away after lunch for a quick power nap to mitigate their afternoon drowsiness.

And some countries have even developed culturally accepted downtimes to combat the natural sluggishness that we feel around midafternoon. In Spain and Italy, people take an afternoon nap—called a *siesta* or *ripòso*—during the sluggish hours. In Chinese cultures, it is common to see workers take a post-lunch nap at their desks. And in Britain and India, many break for tea for a quick caffeine boost in the afternoon.

Our circadian rhythm is under a two-prong influence, one from our body's natural, internal drive, and another from the external cues from the environment—mainly the sun, temperature, etc.

This results in us being more awake around 7 a.m. and 7 p.m., which is why we are more alert during early morning meetings and why television shows clamor for the 7 p.m., prime time slot. They know the science behind our circadian rhythms. Our brains hum to life at this hour, even if they've been sluggish all afternoon.

But if you're experiencing *sleepiness* at 7 a.m. or 7 p.m., the body's naturally active periods, you may be operating with a sleep debt.

Both the internal indicators (homeostatic pressure) and the external cues are important for signaling our brains when it's time to wake up and to fall asleep. Even though this sounds simple, it is a complicated interplay that involves various hormones and chemicals in a precise manner.

If you've ever had to work the night shift or adjust to a different time zone while traveling, for example, you've probably experienced how difficult it can be to self-regulate when your internal and external cues are not in sync with each other.

Let's say you take a flight to Europe. When you arrive, it may be midnight in the time zone where you live but 8 a.m. where you've landed. In this situation, your internal clock will be telling you it's time to sleep, while the environmental cues (sunlight) will be telling you that it's time to wake up. This is why it often takes several days to recover from jet lag, depending on the number of time zones you have crossed.

Hormones that Regulate Sleep and Wakefulness

In addition to internal and external cues, our sleep is also regulated by an array of brain chemicals: some that promote wakefulness and others that help us drift off to sleep. Norepinephrine, dopamine, orexin, cortisol, and histamine are all hormones that our brain releases during the day to keep us awake and alert.

At night, our brains release chemicals like GABA and melatonin to promote sleep. Melatonin is a naturally occurring hormone that induces sleep and makes us feel drowsy, and GABA descends like a fog over the brain, acting as an anesthetic.

These chemicals perform a delicate dance, waxing and waning throughout a 24-hour period to ensure you are awake during the day and asleep at night.

Some non-sleep-related hormones, like human growth hormone (HGH) and testosterone, are also secreted during sleep at varying times during the night. If we don't get enough sleep, we won't get these hormones we need to function during the day.

What *kind* of sleep is just as important as how *much* sleep you get. How you feel the next day depends on the amount of time you spend in stage 3 of non-REM sleep. (If you are tired and groggy despite eight hours of sleep, then you have an issue. You may want to consult a sleep doctor to see if you have a sleep disorder or if your ratio of REM to non-REM sleep is skewed.)

Young, healthy individuals without sleep issues spend roughly 5–15% of their sleep in stage 1, 45–50% in stage 2; 15–20% in stage 3, and 20–25% in REM sleep.

During REM, the brain is still very active, hence it is restless sleep. If you slept eight hours but most of it was in REM sleep or lighter stages of sleep (non-REM stages 1 and 2), it is highly likely you are not well rested.

Some spend most of their sleep in restless REM sleep or have several micro awakenings from sleep disorders like sleep apnea or limb movements and wake up feeling like they never slept.

Stage 3 non-REM, on the other hand, has less cardiovascular variations and is considered the most restful (it is sometimes called sweet sleep). To feel fully rested in the morning, you'll need a fair share of this non-REM sleep to complement your REM sleep.

Until age 20, non-REM slightly predominates, meaning we get more of this sweet sleep than we do REM sleep. As we age, there is more fluctuation with our sleep stages, and stage 3 non-REM sleep is tougher to come by, which is part of the reason sleep strategies become so important.

Certain sleep disorders happen during specific sleep stages. Sleep terrors, sleep talking, and sleepwalking all occur in non-REM sleep, especially in the early part of the night. Sleep apnea, on the other hand, worsens in REM sleep. And nightmares are also more common in REM sleep.

REM behavior disorder (RBD) is a condition predominantly affecting men over 50 and occurs only in REM sleep. With RBD, people physically act out their vivid and sometimes unpleasant dreams.[6]

Barriers to the Natural Sleep Process

Despite how simple it appears on the surface, sleep is a profoundly complex process. As described earlier, your body responds to external stimulation like sunlight and darkness as well as a host of internal hormones and biological processes to regulate sleep rhythms.

As such, there are many factors that can throw our sleep into disarray—stress, natural hormonal changes associated with aging, even the temperature of our bedroom at night. Another way you might inadvertently hinder the flow of your body's production of melatonin is by using electronic devices like phones, computers, TV, and tablets (iPads).

When these devices are used close to bedtime, the light they emit sends signals via your eyes to the brain, informing it that it's still daytime. This way, when you spend a lot of time on electronic devices at night, your brain believes it's still daytime, and it will suppress the release of melatonin, meaning you won't get sleepy.

It's not just the light from devices that encourages wakefulness. Constant access to social media and the news also exacerbates sleep issues by creating stress and anxiety. Your brain naturally scans the horizon for threats to our safety. However, it often cannot tell the difference between a threat that's immediate (like an intruder in your home) and a threat that's distant (like a wildfire 1,000 miles away). For this reason, scrolling late at night or reading the news can send your brain into its fight-or-flight response, even if you're not in imminent danger.

Unfortunately, for many of us, smartphones have become part of our nighttime ritual. We use them to wind down at the end of the day by scrolling mindlessly, not realizing that we're actually making our brain more anxious and alert. Thus, we exert extra pressure on our biology and push away the natural sleep initiation process.

The pandemic amplified this problem. COVID-19-related insomnia became severe for so many people that it earned its own name: Coronasomnia.

Age and life stage can also create hurdles to a good night's sleep. Teenagers, for instance, tend to stay up late, hanging out with friends or spending time on their phones, then go to bed late and wake up late, especially on weekends. This can create an internal clock issue called delayed sleep phase disorder, or circadian rhythm disorder. This happens, in part, because of the teenager's natural physiologic hormonal influences (pubertal hormones) and in part because of societal norms and behavior.

On the other hand, older people (particularly over the age of 70) usually go to bed earlier and wake up earlier, creating the exact opposite problem. We call this advanced sleep phase disorder (ASPD), and it's compounded by the fact the 70-plus population is often retired and prone to take naps during the day. This makes it harder for them to achieve good sleep quality at night.

Sleep is also affected by the ambient temperature. Our bodies fall asleep more easily when the surrounding air is chilly, and I advise my patients to sleep in a room that's slightly below room temperature and experiment with temperatures between 65 and 70 degrees at night. A cooler temperature is also needed for optimal melatonin secretion, thus promoting sleep onset.

It's not surprising that sleep quality is poorer in tropical climates, and it is always better to set temperature at lower level for optimal sleep.

Once our physiology's natural sleep systems have been compromised, we tend to resort to quick fixes and sleep-negative rituals or habits to get better sleep. These bad habits can include using alcohol and over-the-counter sleeping pills to fall asleep at night.

Poor sleep often leads to an increased consumption of caffeine, energy drinks, or sugary products in an effort to boost alertness during the day. In fact, the sale of global energy drinks reached $57.4 billion in 2020 and is expected to grow another 7% by 2025.[7]

Because our brain chemicals are so finely tuned, introducing outside chemicals—even taking a nightly melatonin pill, for example—can be detrimental by *teaching the brain to rely on these outside chemicals rather than producing their own.*

The same goes for chemicals we might take during the day—like caffeine or sugar—to help us wake up. If we interfere too much with our natural orchestra of brain chemistry, our brain may stop producing the chemicals we need for sleeping, and the system is thrown out of balance.

This creates a vicious cycle and is one of the reasons I'm such a big advocate of having healthy sleep strategies *before* problems arise. In these cases, an ounce of prevention is worth *more* than a pound of cure.

Sleep, for Many, Isn't a Priority

"I'll sleep when I'm dead."

"Who needs sleep when there's coffee?"

"I'll catch up on sleep when life calms down."

You've probably heard one or more of these sleep myths being tossed around by bleary-eyed friends and neighbors. Maybe you've even said it yourself.

That's because in today's productivity-obsessed hustle culture, sleep is rarely a priority.

In fact, in some cases, operating on little sleep seems more like a badge of honor when, in reality, it should be a warning sign for what's likely to come. In my practice treating people with sleep issues, I've heard all these myths and more.

Perhaps the most essential biological process next to breathing, sleep is often relegated to the bottom of the vital function totem pole. People talk at length about improving their diet and finally committing to an exercise routine. They buy life-enhancing products, make New Year's resolutions, and join gyms. But I rarely hear about people wanting to make sleep a top priority.

Folks often put off getting help for their sleep issues. They think that because sleep deprivation doesn't progress like cancer and doesn't produce pain like a tooth ache does, they can put off treating it indefinitely. They resolve to patch the problem with a pricy new mattress promising the best sleep of their life, or some new-fangled pillow they saw advertised online.

Or worse, they begin using alcohol to drift off each night and then the next day drink copious amounts of coffee to stay awake. Many people resort to taking sleeping pills, which can lead to a bad habit or even a full-blown addiction.

Unfortunately, these quick fixes just make the underlying problem worse.

Over my many years as a physician, I have come to realize that sleep is just as crucial—perhaps even *more*—than other biological functions. In actuality, sleep is the biological superpower that makes all the other processes possible. It is a complex biological function that helps us process new information, stay healthy, and feel rested. It is essential for growth, concentration, focus, memory, learning, healing, emotional well-being, and more.

If it's that essential, why are so few of us getting the sleep that we need?

An Epidemic of Sleep Deprivation

As modern humans, there are many reasons we try to shortcut on sleep: to get ahead at work, to take night shift work that pays better, or to simply squeeze in one more Facebook post, Instagram reel, or TikTok video.

While modern electronics have allowed us to light up the night, our bodies are not so easy to rewire. Humans are designed to sleep when it's cold, dark, and quiet. If we try to reconfigure our lives so that we stay awake at night or simply don't get a sufficient number of hours of shut eye, our bodies revolt.

As a result, sleep-deprived folks, including second- and third-shift workers, experience higher rates of heart disease,[8] depression, anxiety, type 2 diabetes, and more.[9]

"So, how many hours of sleep do I actually need?"

As a sleep doctor, I hear this question frequently. The answer is that it varies. Most of us need between seven and eight hours of sleep.

But some people, whom I call "short sleepers," can get away with as little as four to six hours with no ill effects, able to function at full mental and physical capacity. But this tends to be a genetic trait and not something most people can engineer, and for most is just not sustainable.

Notoriously short sleeper, Elon Musk, Tesla, SpaceX and Twitter/X CEO refers to himself as "fairly nocturnal."[10] Musk has a history of pulling all-nighters[11] and sleeping under his desk[12] to get work done. But more recently, he has made an effort to sleep at least six hours per night.

"I've tried [to sleep] less, but. . . even though I'm awake more hours, I get less done," Musk told CNBC's David Faber. "And the brain pain level is bad if I get less than six hours [of sleep per night]."

Some highly functioning folks and people in high positions are short sleepers from birth. Several of our previous presidents—including Presidents Obama and Trump—and some corporate executives like Elon Musk are born with this gift. For them, feeling refreshed does not depend on the *quantity* but on the *quality* of sleep.

That said, most of us didn't win the genetic lottery with the short-sleeper trait. If you are sleeping fewer than seven hours and you are still tired, that means you're like the rest of us. You are suffering from insufficient sleep syndrome (ISS). That simply means you *can* sleep, but you are not allowing yourself enough time to get a full night's rest.

And if there were any questions regarding the effects of sleep deprivation, ask any parent of a newborn! Those early days are challenging times until precious little ones are able to sleep through the night.

College-age students or young adults notoriously suffer from ISS. They hardly sleep six hours a night—often due to studying, partying, playing sports, or holding a part-time job—and are chronically sleep-deprived.

I saw my own children become victims of this in their college years. They pushed themselves so hard while they were away at college that when they came home for the week during holidays, they crashed. Sometimes, they slept for 14–16 hours straight to relieve the sleep debt that they incurred over the previous few weeks.

Brandon

I remember my son, Brandon, calling me from campus and stating, "Dad, I think I have a sleep disorder."

"How many hours are you sleeping at night?" I asked.

My son danced around the issue, making all sorts of excuses, and never committing to a firm number. This gave me my answer.

"You don't have a sleep disorder," I told him. "You simply aren't making enough time to sleep."

Just as I suspected, during his next trip home, my son slept more than eight hours a night, wiping out his sleep debt and correcting his sleep schedule.

Unfortunately, it's not just college students who are racking up sleep debts.

More than 40% of adults are sleeping fewer than seven hours.[13] Insufficient sleep is the leading cause of daytime fatigue, and daytime fatigue is a significant cause of poor job performance and work-related accidents. (More about that later.)

Poor sleep is also a contributing factor in various health disorders like high blood pressure, diabetes, obesity, stroke, and even premature death. Poor sleep quality and inadequate sleep does not just affect your physical well-being. Lack of sleep is also correlated with anxiety, depression, and other mood disorders, something we'll look into more in a later chapter.

Statistics tell us that 30–40% of all adults are sleep-deprived,[14] but I would estimate that the numbers are actually much higher. In fact, it's so large a problem that in 2014, the Centers for Disease Control and Prevention (CDC) declared sleep deprivation to be a *public health epidemic* linked to several health issues including hypertension, diabetes, depression, obesity, and cancer.

The sad fact is, when you look at life today, it seems like *nobody's sleeping.*

But why?

In my experience, there are three main causes of sleep deprivation:

- Poor sleep habits
- Underlying physical conditions and sleep disorders
- Unaddressed emotional stress or mental health issues

Poor Sleep Habits

Let's start with sleep hygiene—the medical term for the routines we use to get ready for sleep. This is simply another way of describing our everyday habits or tasks surrounding our sleep. Routines are typically driven by efficiency, convenience, or practicality and can be simple or elaborate.

Whether it's simply changing into pajamas and crawling under the covers or more involved, like doing yoga, listening to music, and drinking sleepy-time tea, we all have some sort of sleep routine.

Many of our routines before bed are adaptive—or sleep-positive routines, as I call them. These include creating a habit of brushing your teeth before you go to bed, taking medications, journaling, meditating or praying, and reading a book just before turning out the light.

But many of us have developed *maladaptive* routines—otherwise known as sleep-negative routines—without even realizing it.

These negative routines can include having a glass or two (or three) of wine, eating fatty or high-carb foods late at night, or scrolling through our social media feeds while in bed. It might be watching an adrenaline-spiking crime show that makes it hard to calm down and surrender to rest.

In today's world of 24/7 news cycles, social media, and geopolitical instability, it's no wonder people find it difficult to unwind at the end of the day. Add that to the problem of constant access created by smartphones, and it's increasingly difficult for folks to get the deep sleep that they need.

Plus, once someone begins having trouble sleeping, it's more likely that they'll develop sleep anxiety, a condition where people feel distressed or afraid to go to bed, as they fear they won't be able to fall asleep. The bedroom soon feels like a torture chamber instead of a place of tranquility and respite.

It's important to note that sleep is not an individual problem to be addressed. Sleep, like healthy lifestyle management, is usually a family affair. If a child isn't sleeping, the parents aren't sleeping. If a spouse isn't sleeping, chances are then their partner usually isn't sleeping either.

The problem is, most of us want to turn sleep on and off with a switch. We want to be scrolling through social media one minute and then fast asleep the next. But as I tell my patients, **initiating sleep is more like using a dimmer switch. You must gradually ease your body into it.**

You wouldn't invite friends over for a dinner party with no preparation. In addition to cooking a lovely meal, you'll set the mood by decorating the table, lighting candles, and turning on some soothing music.

Sleep is similar. You have to prepare well for its arrival, or it may not show up. For many, this means meditating, turning off screens, using white noise, lowering the thermostat, or reading a novel before bed.

Being aware of your sleep habits is one of the first ways to combat the frustrations of poor sleep.

But poor sleep habits aren't the only issue leading to insomnia.

Underlying Physical Conditions and Sleep Disorders

We've all had a restless night's sleep at some time or another, but when you're not able to sleep, it's miserable.

Whether it's an underlying physical problem like chronic pain (like back pain), a tooth ache, or coughing all night because of a bad cold, there are many reasons we lose deep sleep at night.

Other times, the underlying condition is less obvious. Some people may suffer from low iron, which can lead to restless leg syndrome (RLS) causing difficulty initiating sleep.

Similarly, a lack of potassium can lead to a charley horse. If you've ever had such a cramp, you'll know how excruciating it can be and how hard it can be to go back to sleep.

But there is another commonly underdiagnosed condition called sleep apnea. This is when an obstruction or a collapse occurs in the throat or upper airway that causes people to temporarily stop breathing while asleep and causes a drop in oxygen levels.

When your body is deprived of oxygen, the heart must work even harder which, in turn, tends to raise your blood pressure. This stress on the heart then activates the fight-or-flight response.

Untreated sleep disorders can disrupt the body's biorhythms and trigger the release of stress hormones like adrenaline and cortisol, disrupting the body's natural cycles. People with sleep apnea often wake up anxious and alarmed as a result.

Of course, this is not how anyone wants to feel when they wake up in the morning. The goal is to wake up refreshed, energized, and to be able to retain focus throughout the day.

I'll offer more detail later regarding the signs of underlying conditions like sleep apnea and restless legs. I'll also address when to seek help and how you can reduce your risk for these and many other sleep problems.

Unaddressed Emotional Stress or Psychological Issues

Aside from underlying physical problems and poor sleep habits, some sleep deprivation is caused by unaddressed psychological and emotional pain. When a patient comes to see me and I find they have good sleep-positive routines and no underlying health issues yet they're still having trouble sleeping, I often ask about their emotional well-being.

Some people may have an unhealed trauma or loss in their past. Others may lack healthy coping mechanisms for their everyday stresses. In fact, anxiety is a huge reason many people state as causing them not to sleep well.

And when it comes to kids, children are naturally sound sleepers. So, if I see a child with insomnia or who tends to sleep too much, I automatically look for psychological stressors or trauma. Sleep disruptions in children may be a cry for help.

The Benefits of Life-Giving Sound Sleep

Everyone is susceptible to insomnia at various points in our life, whether in our teenage years or in our 70s.

As I mentioned earlier, I had my own struggles during medical school, residency, and fellowship related to working late nights and the pressure to perform. I later found myself struggling to sleep soundly as a small business owner dealing with several major decisions, and also during my grief over the loss of my mom, who was very dear to me.

Instead of relying on quick-fix methods, I resorted to finding long-term practical solutions that have made a significant difference—all for the better. The good news is that as scary as the negative impacts of lack of sleep are, the benefits of healthy sleep are just as amazing.

Good sleep means better memory, focus, mood, energy, immune function, and overall health. Getting the proper amount of sleep can reduce your risk of disease, improve outcomes, help you kick a cold faster, and even improve your resistance to anxiety and depression.

The even better news is that if you aren't a great sleeper now, there are simple steps you can take to transform your sleep so that you wake up feeling refreshed, revitalized, and ready for whatever the day may bring.

Also, my approach has always been to avoid the short-term, pill-mill, quick-fix approach, but rather to work out a long-term permanent solution to sleep issues. The process of creating better and healthier sleep is not always going to be easy, but the results will be fruitful in the long run.

Sound sleep is a *pleasure*. Sleep is free, and it is a necessity for everyone. It is one state where we are all the same, whether you are a king or a commoner. Sleep is the state we all crave and, fortunately, it is there for the taking if you know how to access it.

In the following pages, I'll share with you the impact of various sleep disorders. I'll also share some of the best strategies to help you fall asleep faster, stay asleep longer, and wake up fully rested by the morning.

I'll address

- why we sleep and why we need to sleep;
- effective treatments for sleep issues; and
- the *7 Proven Strategies* to help you sleep better, be more successful, and be happier (and make your family happier).

We spend *a third* of our lives in bed. Isn't it worth the extra effort to make sure that our sleep is deep and nourishing—and that those we live with, and love, can have a better sleep experience as well?

My aim is to give you clear guidelines with the *7 Proven Sleep Strategies* to help you get out of the vicious cycle of poor sleep and the resulting daily exhaustion. When you have effective sleep-positive routines, it will put you back in charge of your life.

I want to do all I can to shed light on this dynamic yet under-appreciated state of rest, restoration, and rejuvenation. Whether your sleep habits need simple tweaking or a full reboot, I'll provide you with a step-by-step guide.

Because when we get a good night's sleep, we can be more productive, energetic, and joyful—and get along better and even live longer.

Transform your sleep, and you'll transform your life.

Chapter 3

Sleep Issues

Insomnia: Not Getting to Sleep, Not Staying Asleep

Kate rolled over and looked at the clock. The orange numbers read 2:49. Inwardly, she wanted to cry.

She had been awake for more than an hour, having gone to bed at midnight so she would be tired enough to go to sleep and *stay* asleep.

But frustratingly, she was wide awake. Again.

She had gotten up once and gone to the family room where it was dark and quiet, only the ticking of the clock making any sound. Occasionally, she would hear the faint rumble of a car driving by.

Kate didn't want to watch TV as she was afraid that it would wake her up even more, so she just sat in her recliner and tried to rest her eyes. She had lost track of how many sleepless nights like this she has endured.

When she couldn't sleep in her chair, she finally gave up and grabbed her phone and started to scroll: Instagram, Facebook, LinkedIn, and TikTok all filled up the small screen.

After an hour of mindless scrolling, she snuck back into the bedroom to try again to sleep, but no matter how hard she tried, the "sleep switch" just wouldn't turn on.

This time, she grabbed her Kindle and picked up where she had left off reading a novel.

When she looked at the clock again, it was 5:25 and in just an hour, it would be time to get up.

Kate continued reading until she could sense the sun coming up.

She got up and set out her clothes and makeup. Hopefully, with some under eye concealer, she wouldn't look as tired as she felt.

The Desolate Night

"I just can't shut off my mind."

"I can't get to sleep."

"I wake up in the middle of the night and can't go back to sleep."

Chronic insomnia can adversely affect health, job stability, and quality of life. Poor work performance, mathematical and technical errors, and motor vehicle accidents are much more common in people with chronic insomnia. In fact, those with insomnia have also been shown to be twice as likely to be in a car wreck.[15]

Persistent insomnia has also been identified in multiple studies as a significant risk factor for the development of psychiatric disorders, especially mood disorders, and can exacerbate anxiety and depressive symptoms. Folks with insomnia stay awake longer and tend to eat more; hence they are at a higher risk of obesity, and an increased risk for hypertension and cardiovascular disease.

Sleep deprivation and poor sleep quality can have harmful effects and make us susceptible to several other medical conditions. People who sleep fewer than 6 hours have a higher mortality rate than those who sleep 7–9 hours.[16] That's because lack of sleep affects all organs, contributing to high blood pressure, stroke, diabetes, heart issues, and also affecting our mental health.

Sleep hygiene and good sleep discipline are necessary for better health and for safety in general.

How Did We Get Here?

Before the Industrial Revolution, the general public slept for as many as 14 hours a night. They went to bed when the sun set and woke up when it rose again. That meant that in the winter, when nights were long and days were short, people spent huge portions of time asleep, so much so that some historians even believe that biphasic sleep—sleeping in two long periods separated by a short period of wakefulness—was common.[17]

Unfortunately, as more and more homes got electricity, people could carry on with their activities later into the night as lightbulbs were much more powerful than candles. This resulted in people spending less time in bed. But even when they'd go to bed, it was now harder to fall asleep due to our brains being so sensitive to light.

Fast forward to 2014, and the CDC announced that sleep deprivation has become a full-blown epidemic. In fact, a study on insomnia between 1993 and 2015 found that the "diagnosis of insomnia during office visits in the United States increased elevenfold, from 800,000 to 9.4 million."[18]

What's more, in 2020, The National Sleep Foundation's "Sleep in America" poll found that "Americans feel sleepy on an average of three days a week, with many saying it impacts their daily activities, mood, mental acuity, productivity and more."[19] Many people are seeking over-the-counter help instead of speaking with their physician.

Visit your local drug store, and you'll find rows upon rows of sleep aids and commercial products, such as gummies, hot cocoa mixes, sleepy-time teas, and more. Want to stay cool at night? You can now buy a mattress topper with a climate control remote that promises "more restorative sleep."

There are even companies selling cookies that cater to folks who cannot sleep by delivering cookies until 3 a.m. (Not that those would make you sleep.)

Despite all these fancy options designed to help us sleep—or at least to get us to spend more in the *hopes* we will sleep better—people today are sleeping worse than ever. Consequently, the prevalence of insomnia has increased significantly over the years.

I often tell my patients that the bedroom should be reserved only for sex and sleeping, but sadly, many people use this space as an extension of their offices and bring their laptops and paperwork to bed. Others view the bedroom as an extension of their living room, watching TV while in bed until the early morning hours.

Without setting clear boundaries around what the bedroom should and should not be used for, it's easy to see how this space loses its peaceful and calming allure.

My patients lament that their rooms have become crucibles of worry and stress, and that they lie in bed ruminating on the events of the day. That's because many of them are suffering from insomnia, a disorder that causes persistently poor sleep or lack of sleep.

Unlike other disorders, it's hard to identify one specific biological cause for this ailment. Insomnia is often a result of our maladaptive bedtime habits, or the lack of good sleep strategies. Insomnia could also result from medical and psychiatric conditions.

The Prevalence of Insomnia

According to the CDC, an estimated 83.6 million adults in the US sleep fewer than seven hours per night.[20] Of those, about 30–40% of individuals report occasional nighttime insomnia.[21] The rate of chronic insomnia hovers around 10–15%.[22] Even more concerning, around 40% of American adults report that they've accidentally fallen asleep during the day.[23]

Stress and worry are some of the most common factors for poor quality of sleep. Young children, who are typically great sleepers, may experience occasional insomnia due to the stresses of peer pressure, examinations, bullying, or from excessive screen time before bed.

The largest gap between recommended and actual sleep deprivation is in the 14–17 age group, where the recommended sleep time is 8–10 hours while the actual sleep time 6–7 hours.

Insomnia in adults is often triggered by constant worry and our inability to tune our mind out.

However, as common as insomnia is today, most of it goes undiagnosed, in part because insomnia can masquerade as other health issues. It can look like general fatigue, depression, anxiety, or even attention-deficit/hyperactivity disorder (ADHD). Therefore, it is important to address sleep issues routinely during wellness visits with your family physician.

What Is Insomnia?

So, how is insomnia different from old fashioned sleeplessness? The *Diagnostic and Statistical Manual of Mental Disorders, Fifth Edition* (DSM-5) defines insomnia as the difficulty initiating and maintaining sleep, "characterized by frequent awakenings or problems returning to sleep after awakenings."[24]

Insomnia has an ongoing impact on both nights and days, with a difficulty of falling asleep and maintaining sleep, as well as experiencing clinically significant distress in multiple areas of life.[25]

Insomnia is characterized by persistent dissatisfaction with sleep quantity or quality, by specific complaints of difficulty falling asleep, by frequent nighttime awakenings, and by difficulty returning to sleep. It's also often associated with awakenings earlier in the morning than desired.

In addition, insomnia may be characterized by significant distress or impairment in daytime functioning, as indicated by symptoms such as fatigue, daytime sleepiness, impairment in cognitive performance, and mood disturbances.[26] Untreated insomnia is associated with significant consequences and comorbidities, including psychological, physical, and occupational impairment as well as a significant economic burden.[27]

It is important to rule out other sleep disorders, especially sleep apnea, which can be the single-most treatable cause of poor sleep and insomnia, as these can coexist.

Sleep apnea affects sleep quality because the episodes of stopping breathing at night can lead to awakenings. This results in awakenings and creates an inability to go back to sleep. Other sleep disorders, like periodic limb movements at night, can also result in frequent awakenings at night.

What Causes Insomnia?

When someone doesn't sleep well, the goal is to determine whether they have a primary *sleep* disorder—meaning they do not have a *medical* or *mental* disorder causing them not to sleep—or if they have a case of clear-cut insomnia. They may have conditions like sleep apnea, RLS, limb movement disorders, or clock issues (like circadian rhythm disorders) that can affect their sleep.

Teasing out a specific cause for ongoing insomnia is tricky because everyone experiences sleeplessness at some point in their lives, whether it's due to a loss, trauma, or stress related to work.

So, why do some people develop insomnia while others return to healthy sleep habits once the event has ended? Unlike other sleep disorders, insomnia is more subjective, rather than a solely physiological problem.

When insomnia *does* become a chronic problem, it's generally because the person compounds the problem by introducing bad sleep habits or quick fixes that are harmful in the long run. Some people follow good sleep hygiene and still have insomnia. Typically, I proceed by using a process of elimination when trying to reach the bottom of a person's chronic insomnia.

If the person has other medical conditions like heart, lung, or emotional problems contributing to their insomnia, of course those need to be addressed and resolved first. Once those are eliminated, it's important to investigate the routines that they have been practicing. Often, these have a negative impact on their sleep, even though they're using them in an effort to sleep better.

The most famous routine is "counting sheep" to try and induce sleep. This is fundamentally flawed as the process of counting causes increases cognitive activity, which is counterproductive to initiating sleep.

The easiest way to understand the causes of insomnia is to divide them into three categories:

- Predisposing (increasing the likelihood)
- Precipitating (causing)
- Perpetuating (continuing)

Predisposing factors include anything that makes us more susceptible to insomnia, including gender, age, and family history. These can't be changed, but they can be managed.

For example, women are naturally inclined to poor sleep due to hormonal changes and from having to be hyper vigilant in their role as caregivers. Because of this heightened awakening state, women have a significantly higher incidence of insomnia.

Sleep also becomes more difficult to attain as we age due to changes in the brain. In addition, genetics plays a role in how well we sleep—other family members could also suffer with insomnia.

When it comes to predisposing factors (like life circumstances), you may not have a choice in the matter, but you can choose what you do with it. Even though some people will always be more predisposed to insomnia, they can implement good sleep strategies that mitigate these factors and help them achieve the best rest possible.

Precipitating factors include life-changing events like the death of a loved one, a divorce, or the loss of a job. These events can be abrupt and unexpected, and they naturally cause us to lose sleep. But the effect is usually temporary.

Most insomnia triggered by precipitating events—even major events—resolve within six months, but sometimes the effects can linger. Like with predisposing factors, these events cannot be controlled, but we can choose how we respond to these events so that they don't create permanent sleep issues.

Other times, a precipitating factor can be as simple as having a flight the next day. Some people sleep poorly the night before a flight because they're worried that they will miss their plane.

For others, the anxiety of preparing for and taking an exam can lead to a lack of sleep. Test anxiety is prevalent among high schoolers and college-aged students, and I personally used to suffer from this during high school and college. I used to get so worked up about exams that my sleep quality was poor the night before I took them.

Lack of sleep leads to more anxiety, and anxiety leads to poor sleep. Poor sleep can also lead to poor memory, which is not at all helpful if you're about to take an exam.

I learned through my experience how damaging this negative loop can be. No amount of preparation was sufficient; I couldn't shut my mind down enough to get restful sleep. Eventually, I realized I needed to find a solution since exam preparation was going to be a forever phenomenon in the medical field.

Unfortunately, in the 1980s when I was in med school, there was not much information available about how to deal with my sleeplessness. Back then, insomnia wasn't much of a buzz word, and my peers weren't openly talking about their sleep issues. However, med school is so academically rigorous and competitive that I knew I wasn't the only one losing sleep to cram in more study time. So, I set out to figure out how to insomnia-proof myself.

The first step was adequate preparation for the exams, which I was already doing. Then, as the dates for the exams were nearing, I had to find a way to calm myself so I could sleep better. I achieved this by sticking to a strict schedule and easing into bed at a fixed time every night. But when med school—and my subsequent residency and fellowship—necessarily included variable schedules, this was tough to do, but I stuck to my set bedtime as much as possible.

I also started reading fiction and *other* books—nothing too scary, mostly books with a quick-moving plot that captured my attention—prior to sleep. I also used my imagination to create story lines, a technique I call Vivid Imagination®. To this day I still use it to fall asleep.

I also started to limit my coffee intake, which I must admit was hard to do because I had to stay up late to prepare for exams. At the time, I was not fully aware that the effects of caffeine can last up to 12 hours, but I could tell that restricting my coffee intake helped me sleep better.

By performing these routines consistently for several weeks, I was able to remove the anxiety and the habit of getting worked up prior to examinations.

In my 40s when my mom passed away, I dealt with another bout of insomnia, this time related to grief. Everyone deals with grief differently, but one of the most common features is the inability to sleep. The initial shock of losing a loved one along with the aftermath of the void can be overwhelming, and there is nothing one can do about this. It can last a few days to weeks.

In my case, even months after my mother passed, I had waves of emotions leading to poor sleep. It was then that I decided I had to change my reaction to this loss. I had to come to terms with my grief and decide to move forward.

Long before my mother passed away, I had planned to go on a mission trip. In the midst of my grief, I decided I would still participate. Doing something physically strenuous helped get my mind off my loss. The timing of the mission trip may have been a coincidence, but it helped me take my mind off the vicious cycle of bereavement and sleep loss and make a fresh start. I'm so grateful that it gave me the chance to break my routine.

Joining a sports team or trying a new hobby are other good ways to change up your routine so that grief becomes less acute. I recommend this strategy to many of my patients who are in a rut: take a break and then make a fresh start.

But while it is OK to take a break from grief and stress, it is also important to process the grief. Once this is addressed, I recommend implementing my *7 Proven Sleep Strategies* to get back on track. Many of my patients suffer from grief-related insomnia, and my own experience with it helps me empathize with their pain and helps them know that the intensity of grief will diminish over time.

Perpetuating factors are the most notorious and hard to shake. Folks get in a rut with a bad habit and cannot seem to break it. People often ruminate and spend time and energy focusing on *not* sleeping, which only reinforces the issues that got them there in the first place. They start worrying and feel they cannot wind down. This feeds their anxiety, and often bleeds over into the bedroom, resulting in an inability to go to sleep.

This learned behavior is usually years in the making, mainly due to misinformation they had gathered in an effort to self-heal. This results in self-imposed sleep routines that result in poorer sleep.

These routines may include watching TV in bed, playing games on their personal devices, using lights and scented candles, and on and on. People also try alcohol, over-the-counter medications, marijuana, and sometimes prescription medications. These often help for a while but not on a long-term, sustainable basis. And for those who rely on prescription sleep meds, it often leads to a dependence on the medication, known as hypnotic dependent insomnia.

When we give into quick fixes or bad habits or routines, we surrender our body's natural power to induce sleep without external help. Additionally, many of these habits can leave us feeling groggy—even dizzy—the next morning. This can result in falls and other accidents.

Unfortunately, many people don't share this information with their doctors, so it's hard to pinpoint how often this occurs. However, in my practice, I've seen it all too often.

People tend to already know that sleep aids cause drowsiness, so you shouldn't take them if you're planning to drive. Additionally, people sometimes combine alcohol and sedatives or pain medications to help their sleep. These behaviors can result in dangerous outcomes.

Stress and Insomnia

Stress plays a major role in affecting the quality of sleep. When talking to patients, I try to identify the causes of their stressors and guide them to get help in that area. These stressors could be either physical, mental, or psychological. (The way I think of it, mental stressors are more analytical, visual, and belief centered. Psychological stressors are our emotions and fears.)

Rachael

My twenty-two-year-old daughter, Rachael, recently experienced a time with very poor quality of sleep. She was in her final year of college and had been stressing about which law school she would choose. By the time Rachael called me, she hadn't been sleeping well for three months. She had googled *insomnia* and tried several strategies, including a white noise machine, meditation music, and melatonin.

Rachael didn't talk to me about this earlier as she knew I usually don't treat family members, even for something as simple as a sore throat—I tell them to see their personal physician. But when she finally talked to me about her sleep problem, I wanted to help her, of course.

When I asked her about her sleep routines, Rachael told me she tried to go to sleep between 10:30 and 11 p.m., but she had been spending many evenings working late on her law-school applications. And when it was time to go to sleep, she sometimes had a hard time winding down and shutting off her mind.

Rachael also told me that she often woke up in the middle of the night, and when she woke up, she'd look at her watch or phone, which seemed to make things worse.

We talked about how increased cognitive activity prior to sleep is the number-one cause of not being able to fall asleep immediately, as it's natural for the mind to be still thinking about all the possibilities of the decisions you have to make. I asked her to leave the phone and other electronic devices beyond reach from her bed. I also asked her to set an alarm clock for her desired wake-up time.

Rachael mentioned that to stay focused, she would often drink a macchiato around 7 p.m. I strongly discouraged her habit of drinking caffeinated beverages past 4 p.m. Not only is caffeine a stimulant, it also acts as a diuretic, which had resulted in some of her nightly awakenings.

Finally, I asked my daughter to log her sleep using the Sleep Journal I often have my patients fill out. (You can find the Sleep Journal and Sleep Assessment at the back of this book or download them from SleepFixAcademy.com.)

Not long after, Rachael called me again. "Dad, you are the best sleep doctor in the world!" she declared. As parents, we are well aware that our children don't necessarily give us any credit, so I was over the moon when she complimented me.

Fortunately, she had only struggled with this schedule for three months, and within two weeks of following the strategies, she was able to get back on track. I discussed with her how when you want to be successful in life and make good decisions—especially as a lawyer—sound sleep hygiene and a good restful sleep are non-negotiables.

Rachael was feeling so much better that she shared the information with several friends, who then made changes and were also feeling better. To me, this further fueled my passion to get this information out to help many more young adults and others suffering from insomnia.

Insomnia and Comorbidities

Insomnia often can coexist with several psychological, medical, and sleep disorders. The simultaneous presentation of insomnia and another condition was historically termed *secondary insomnia*, meaning a psychiatric or medical disorder was the *cause* of the insomnia.

The term has been replaced with *comorbid insomnia* in DSM-5, meaning that insomnia can coexist with other disorders, not just as the cause or the effect. This change also highlights the recognition that insomnia can be a contributor to other psychological and medical disorders rather than simply being a symptom of these conditions.

If insomnia occurs concurrently with sleep apnea, it is called COMISA (comorbid insomnia with sleep apnea).

The medical term *comorbidity* refers to the presence of two or more diseases or medical conditions at the same time. It also recognizes the importance of attending to both insomnia and the comorbid condition during treatment. This change in classification also acknowledges that the causal relationship between psychiatric disorders and insomnia is more complex than researchers previously believed.

For those struggling with insomnia, it can be *miserable*.

I often liken it to having a small, smoldering fire of wakefulness. Old-school approaches to insomnia are akin to dropping fire-retardant chemicals with a helicopter to try and put out the small fire. In this way, many of the medications used to treat insomnia affect the entire brain, leaving patients groggy the next day.

Fortunately, there is great interest and research in treatments used to target the areas of the brain that are specific to wakefulness, thus resulting in fewer side effects and better sleep.

Pain and Insomnia

Pain is one of the main medical causes of comorbid insomnia.

Pain is a physical form of stress that can be easily identified, and appropriate treatment results in a return to restorative sleep. Physical pain is often a perpetuating factor that affects sleep, meaning while it didn't necessarily cause insomnia, pain often disrupts consolidated sleep.

The source of pain can be the result of medical conditions like diabetic neuropathy, or issues with arthritis, or back pain related to degenerative disc disease. Sleeping in certain positions can also aggravate the pain, and, in turn, affect the quality of sleep.

Your first line of defense to alleviate pain could be natural options, like physical therapy, massage, yoga, and chiropractic and acupuncture therapies. These therapies often result in significant improvement in pain. A consultation with a primary care provider can help to guide therapy and treatment.

Once the source of chronic pain is identified and treated, it is easier to rest.

Sleep Apnea: The "Not So Silent" Silent Killer

Peggy thought she was going to totally lose her mind. She and John had been married for 42 years and they had finally come into their empty-nest years. The kids were grown and off, and the couple was awaiting the birth of their first grandchild.

But Peggy was *exhausted*. At first, John's snoring was mildly irritating. But over time, it had gotten steadily worse.

She had tried prodding him with her elbow in the middle of the night. Often that worked. Once he moved or turned over, he would stop snoring.

As of late, he was snoring so loud at night that it woke her up from a sound sleep. And even if she pushed and prodded, he was quickly back to snoring so loud she couldn't go back to sleep. (Her not sleeping is called environmental sleep disorder, meaning she couldn't sleep on account of her spouse's snoring).

But the part that was really driving Peggy nuts was that John was clueless.

He thought he was "just fine." He was conscientious about what he ate, worked out at the gym every day, and maintained a healthy weight.

Peggy had tried convincing him that he needed to get help (he perceived it as nagging, and there may have been a bit of truth to that), but he just didn't think it was necessary, not to mention that he thought the testing was a pain and too complex.

After a while, Peggy declared that she had had enough, and she gave John an ultimatum: If he didn't address his snoring issue, they would be getting a *sleep divorce*, meaning he would have to sleep in the guest bedroom. The sheets were clean and ready for him.

She was serious and he knew it. Like many spouses do, Peggy made a recording of his snoring and emailed him the name of a sleep doctor. John was finally forced to take his snoring seriously. He called the clinic the next morning to make an appointment just to make his wife happy and get her off his back. He was convinced a sleep study would vindicate him.

Needless to say, he was shocked when his in-home study showed that he had 35 episodes of sleep apnea per hour, where he actually stopped breathing.

The data didn't lie.

He got fitted with a CPAP and started using it immediately.

Since a CPAP machine prevents you from snoring, the very first night he used it, he didn't snore. Peggy got her first good night's sleep in ages and woke up refreshed.

She was relieved on two levels: She was finally able to sleep peacefully, and she knew John was getting the treatment he needed so he wasn't putting so much pressure on his heart and vital organs. She really wanted him to stay around so they could enjoy their golden years and have the life they had always planned.

As for John, well, he never admitted the CPAP made a difference. But he kept using it and never missed a night.

It was obvious to Peggy that it made him feel better or he never would have continued to use it.

Sometimes, actions speak louder than words.

If you've ever been irritated at the sound of someone snoring, you know it can be loud. Unfortunately, when people are sleeping, they don't hear themselves snore.

Snoring is the sound that occurs due to the vibration of tissue in the throat due to air going through a narrow passage. The main culprit is the tongue and the soft palate falling back into the throat and causing an obstruction, either partial or complete.

As the air goes through the obstructed pathway, the surrounding tissues vibrate, causing sounds of various decibels depending on the degree of obstruction.

Snoring is louder in men due to their larger size creating a longer airway and larger voice box (larynx), thus amplifying the sound.

Though the term *sleep apnea* was only introduced in the 1960s, the problem has existed throughout history. If you look closely, you can find the symptoms of sleep apnea—loud snoring and the interruption of breath during sleep—showing up in all kinds of historical texts.

The Greek god Dionysus was said to snore so loudly he would ask the women surrounding him to poke him with his own rod to wake him up when he stopped breathing.

Sleep apnea also appeared in Charles Dicken's novel *The Pickwick Papers*. Dickens described a boy named Joe who also snored and woke up abruptly, likely from a lack of oxygen. Because of this description, physicians referred to this group of symptoms as Pickwickian syndrome for many years.

It wasn't until 1965 that doctors discovered the root cause of these symptoms—the repeated cessation of breathing during sleep, whether caused by a physical obstruction or the suppression of the respiratory system—and coined the term *sleep apnea*. Apnea is derived from Greek word *apnoia* meaning without breath or the absence of breathing.

There are several medical disorders that tend to creep up as we age, like diabetes, hypertension, heart, and memory issues. For many people, sleep apnea is the common denominator in all these issues. That means when sleep apnea is properly treated and managed, it can improve a host of other problems.

Today, 30 million Americans are affected by sleep apnea, of which 80% are still undiagnosed, costing the country more than $149 billion annually in health care costs, lost work productivity, and workplace and motor vehicle accidents.[28] It's clear that both the physical and economic impact on our lives from sleep apnea are tremendous.

There are three types of sleep apnea:

- Obstructive sleep apnea, which is the most common, accounts for 95% of all sleep apnea cases.
- Central sleep apnea, caused by suppression of the breathing center in the brain, accounts for 1–5% of cases and is mostly due to narcotic medications or due to CPAP treatment, i.e., it is treatment induced.
- Mixed sleep apnea, a combination of obstructive and central sleep apnea, accounts to 2–3% of total incidents of sleep apnea.

Obstructive sleep apnea (or OSA, a term you'll find throughout this book) is caused by either a partial or complete collapse of the airway. When there is a complete cessation of air flow, this is called apnea. And when there is partial cessation, it's called hypopnea.

The chest muscles and diaphragm work hard to open the airway, sometimes causing a loud gasp or body jerk to wake the person—and their spouse or partner! The person may not be fully awake, but brain wave activity would indicate there are micro awakenings prompting them to take their next breath. This happens several times at night, causing folks not to get restful sleep. They wake up the next day feeling tired.

The apnea hypopnea index (AHI) is a term commonly used when reporting the number of apnea and hypopnea episodes per hour. The severity of sleep apnea is reported as mild if the events occur 5–14 times per hour, moderate for 15–29 events, and severe for 30 or more episodes per hour.

These episodes can happen in different sleep stages. However, in REM sleep, the muscles are paralyzed, making folks more vulnerable.

Sam

Sam was a financially successful building contractor but an unhappy man. Over time—especially during the pandemic—he had packed on the pounds, weighing in at more than 350 pounds. At his annual checkup with his primary care physician, Sam admitted he was tired of being physically uncomfortable. (He said he was having trouble getting in and out of chairs, cars, and always having to ask for the seatbelt extender on an airplane.) Sam looked quite despondent and said it was finally time to do *something*—though he didn't know what.

Just 53 years old, Sam had high blood pressure and diabetes. He snored loudly, and his wife, Andrea, told him she was concerned because she had noticed him stop breathing multiple times at night. He had been living with these many problems for over 10 years.

As he had done in the past, Sam's doctor highly recommended that Sam get a sleep study. Although Sam didn't like the idea of in-lab testing where he would be watched by strangers, he told his doctor he was finally willing to do whatever it took to feel better.

When Sam came to my office for his appointment, even though he took the elevator, he was short of breath. His diabetes was off the charts and his blood pressure was extremely elevated. His feet were swollen up to his knees. He had been recently admitted to the hospital and was found to be in right and left-sided heart failure and fluid overload.

Because of his size and the complexity of his medical conditions, I would have sent him for an in-lab sleep study, but due to COVID, the earliest availability to do the testing was three weeks away. When I suggested a home-based study for the very same day, Sam was visibly relieved not to have to go to the hospital.

The next morning, when he returned his sleep study device, I wasn't at all surprised it showed severe sleep apnea with an AHI of 70 episodes *per hour*.

Because of the severity of Sam's medical problems, I prescribed a CPAP machine with a rush order. Unfortunately, there was a delay in getting him the CPAP due to a massive recall of one model and supply-chain issues due to the pandemic.

What normally takes two weeks was going to take 3–6 months.

The medical-supply company was doing everything they could to get him a machine as soon as possible. But sadly, before Sam could get the CPAP, he was found unresponsive at his house one morning. Andrea tried to revive him and paramedics performed CPR, but it was in vain. He died en route to the hospital. Untreated severe sleep apnea contributed to his heart failure, which likely triggered heart arrhythmia and resulted in sudden cardiac arrest.

Unfortunately, Sam isn't the only person whose death has been attributed to sleep apnea. All-American professional football player Reggie White[29] and famous Indian singer Bappi Lahiri have been reported to have died from complications of sleep apnea.[30]

Risk Factors for Sleep Apnea

Sleep apnea can occur at all ages, and I've treated children as young as three years old. That said, it's typically more common in middle age and old age. It is also more prevalent in men than women since hormones like estrogen and progesterone naturally offer some protection against sleep apnea, but prevalence increases with age, especially after menopause.

When there is a lack of oxygen, estrogen and progesterone act as respiratory stimulants. They also help reduce the oxidative stress on the upper airway, thus lowering the risk of an oropharyngeal (upper airway) collapse. In women, once estrogen levels drop with menopause, tissues around the throat lose their tonicity and become more flaccid, causing an obstruction.

A study in Wisconsin revealed post-menopausal women have a 3.5 times higher risk of sleep apnea compared to premenopausal women.[31] There is also an increased incidence of sleep apnea in women who have polycystic ovarian disease due to weight gain and hormonal changes.

Aside from hormones, there are other reasons that women are diagnosed with sleep apnea less often than men, namely, women do not show the classic symptoms like loud snoring, and women are less likely to report snoring.

Sleep apnea rates also vary with race, with a higher incidence of sleep apnea in young African American and South Asian men due to differences in the anatomy of the airway and other risk factors.[32,33]

Common Causes of Sleep Apnea

Weight gain and obesity are some of the biggest risk factors for sleep apnea. Weight is uniformly distributed around the body, including in the soft tissues of the throat. This additional weight creates pressure on the neck, which can cause an obstruction to the natural flow of air.

An enlarged neck circumference—over 17 inches in men and 16 inches in women—predisposes people to OSA.[34] Losing weight can help with mild and moderate sleep apnea, but severe apnea requires more involved treatment.

Enlarged tonsils and adenoids are especially common in children and can create an obstruction. For children, surgically removing the tonsils and adenoids can usually fully resolve or significantly improve sleep apnea.

The position of the jaw can also cause an obstruction. For people with an overbite, for example, the jaw is pushed backward, causing obstruction.

Abnormalities of the nose, including a deviated nasal septum, nasal polyps, and the enlargement of the nasal tissue (called turbinate hypertrophy) can all cause nasal-passage obstruction, hence blocking air flow.

Thyroid abnormalities. The thyroid gland produces thyroid hormone that affects metabolism. It can cause muscle and tissue changes. When the hormone levels are too low, the result is a thyroid hormone surge, which causes enlargement in the tongue and surrounding tissues, resulting in a narrowing of the throat area.

Smoking provokes inflammation of the upper airways, which can narrow the air passages. Marijuana, when smoked, also causes airway inflammation and can slow down the respiratory system.

Narcotic pain medication, i.e., opioids, can cause apnea by depressing the respiratory center in the brain, causing the respiratory center to become lazy and making the breath slower and shallower.

Body position while sleeping can also predispose people to an obstruction, especially when sleeping on the back as gravity pushes the tongue and the surrounding tissues backward causing the obstruction.

Birth defects and deformities such as facial, palatal, and cranial abnormalities can cause structural obstruction. Facial abnormalities, as seen in patients with Down syndrome, predisposes them to obstruction.

Alcohol causes relaxation of the throat muscles and tongue, thus causing an obstruction. In addition to creating this physical obstruction, alcohol also slows down the respiratory center in the brain, making people more at risk for episodes of apnea.

Genetics also plays a part, as obstructive sleep apnea can be inherited.

Sleep Apnea and Cognitive Health

Sleep apnea places folks at a high risk for dementia. Scientists believe this is because the lack of oxygen during an apnea episode leads to inflammatory changes and a narrowing in the smaller blood vessels supplying oxygen to the brain. Years of low oxygen in the blood (hypoxemia) to the brain can lead to irreversible brain damage, especially to the areas of the brain associated with cognition and memory.

One study found that people with sleep apnea-related hypoxemia had more severe cognitive impairment than those who had sleep apnea without hypoxemia.[35] Those with hypoxemia also scored lower on a series of cognitive tests. This suggests that the lack of oxygen associated with sleep apnea is a significant contributor to cognitive decline.

The root cause of Alzheimer's disease and dementia is still unknown, but sleep apnea can exacerbate both conditions. Sleep apnea also makes it harder for the brain to activate the glymphatic system and clean itself each night. If a person can't sleep, the brain won't have a chance to self-cleanse. When that happens, the brain becomes less able to function properly.

A 2022 study looked at how sleep apnea affected white matter and cognition in the brain over a four-year period.[36] People with persistent OSA showed the biggest declines in their white matter integrity, and these changes were proven with cognitive tests.

People with mild sleep apnea, on the other hand, had *some* white matter changes, but theirs were not as significant as people with severe OSA. Participants who had previously experienced OSA, but who had resolved it through treatment, scored better than their peers on visual recall and immediate recall tests.[37,38]

These findings suggest that treating OSA early can prevent cognitive decline and preserve brain function.

The severity of damage also depends on the severity of sleep apnea. Sleep apnea is classified as mild, moderate, or severe depending on the total number of episodes of apneas (stopping breathing) and hypopneas (partial closure) that occur per hour. (As you may recall, this is referred to as the apnea hypopnea index, or AHI.)

When the AHI is between 5 and 14, it is considered mild, 15–29 is moderate, and over 30 is considered severe. The more severe the sleep apnea, and more prolonged the duration of low oxygen, the higher the chance of irreversible damage to the brain.[39]

Joe

Joe was a 43-year-old, fairly fit, marketing and sales executive who reluctantly came to my office after his wife complained of severe snoring. She had also noticed interrupted breathing in his sleep, especially on nights he drank. He was a heavy drinker who would have at least three or four glasses of whiskey five nights a week. This was back in 2007 when the practice of the home sleep study was not available, so I sent him to an in-lab study.

Two days prior to his test, Joe called my office and wanted to know if he could bring his alcohol and some snacks to the testing site. Obviously, I said no to the alcohol and yes to the snacks.

As expected, since he didn't drink his evening whiskey on the night of the study, he didn't have significant apnea events that night.

A few years later, he heard that home sleep apnea testing was readily available, and (with the encouragement of his wife) Joe decided to get retested to prove to his wife he was still fine. He was astounded when I reviewed his study, which showed that he had severe sleep apnea. Joe was treated with CPAP.

Once he was confronted with the impact of alcohol on his breathing and sleeping, Joe decided to cut back on his drinking. And once he quit drinking entirely, his apnea improved significantly.

Common Symptoms of Sleep Apnea

- Snoring due to air moving through a narrow passage, creating vibrations
- Being tired, excessive daytime fatigue, and a lack of energy due to repeated awakenings from apnea episodes

- Stopping breathing and sleep pauses. A partner often notices the pause in breathing, then nudges the person to wake up to kickstart the breathing
- Moodiness and irritability due to a lack of quality sleep
- Dry mouth due to mouth breathing to try and catch a breath
- Sore throat from the effects of snoring
- Sensation of choking, gasping, and interrupted breathing from the body's struggle to breathe
- Sexual dysfunction. Severe untreated sleep apnea is associated with low testosterone levels due to the lack of oxygen supply to the sex organs. It can also contribute to low sperm count, infertility, relationship challenges, and a lack of libido due to fatigue
- Cognitive dysfunction, including a lack of clarity and brain fog due to repeated awakenings
- Frequent urination due to the heart secreting hormones to get rid of excess fluid
- Frequent headaches, especially in the mornings, due to blood vessels stretching to deliver oxygen
- Worsening of anxiety and depression due to poor quality of sleep
- For children, bedwetting, learning disabilities like ADHD, along with poor school performance due to lack of good sleep
- Excessive night sweats due to excess effort to breathe
- Teeth grinding, jaw soreness, and tooth damage
- Sudden cardiac death. Apnea can place the heart under stress and can provoke arrhythmia, resulting in sudden cardiac death

How Sleep Apnea Stresses the Body

Untreated, the stress of sleep apnea on the body can cause a cascade of other health issues. As the air travels the obstructed pathway, the flow sensors that are strategically placed along the throat sense the lack of air flow. When interruption of the breath occurs, the resultant buildup of carbon dioxide triggers a flight-or-fight response that causes awakenings. Even though you think you are sleeping eight or more hours, it is not of good quality as you are woken up multiple times a night due to the occurrence of apnea.

This flight-or-fight response releases stress hormones like norepinephrine. This causes high blood pressure, which, in turn, causes stress on the heart, adding to the risk of stroke and heart attacks. High norepinephrine can also cause problems controlling blood sugar (diabetes) and heart rhythm issues (like atrial fibrillation).

Blood pressure is supposed to be lower at night, thus creating an equilibrium and a chance for the cardiovascular system to rest. However, apnea prevents this stabilization from happening due to the release of stress hormones. Thus, the body does not get a chance to heal, and blood pressure tends to be higher and more difficult to control in people with sleep apnea.

Primary care physicians are aware of the causal effects of blood pressure due to sleep apnea, and they often tend to refer folks to me for this reason.

Low libido caused by low testosterone is also a common reason for referral to my practice. Severe sleep apnea is often associated with low testosterone levels due to the lack of oxygen supply to the testes.

Women with sleep apnea also struggle more with infertility than women who sleep well. In a 2021 study conducted in Taiwan, women with OSA had twice the risk of female infertility compared to women who have never had sleep apnea.[40] (I'll discuss the relationship between sex and sleep issues in more detail later.)

Repeated awakenings due to apnea can worsen the quality of sleep, and this can worsen anxiety and depressive symptoms. Poor sleep quality affects workplace performance, and sleep-deprived individuals are prone to cause more errors, as mentioned in chapter one.

Multiple apnea episodes often result in hypoxia, or low blood oxygen, which leads to damage to multiple organs, especially the brain. At first, this problem manifests as simple brain fog or drowsiness. If left untreated, several years of apnea can lead to irreversible and permanent damage to memory and cognitive function.

Thus, for any person who has been newly diagnosed with high blood pressure or has memory or concentration issues, a sleep evaluation needs to be considered to rule out sleep apnea. If there are heart issues or difficulty controlling blood sugar, and if they have other risk factors like obesity, folks should also ask to have a sleep study conducted.

People who have a breathing disorder called emphysema (also known as chronic obstructive pulmonary disorder, or COPD) can also have obstructive sleep apnea—a phenomenon called overlap syndrome. Treatment with CPAP often improves both breathing and sleep apnea problems.

Apnea in young children is associated with behavioral and attention-deficit disorder. The symptoms of sleep apnea in children are subtle. (For more information, refer to Chapter 8 for sleep disorders in children.)

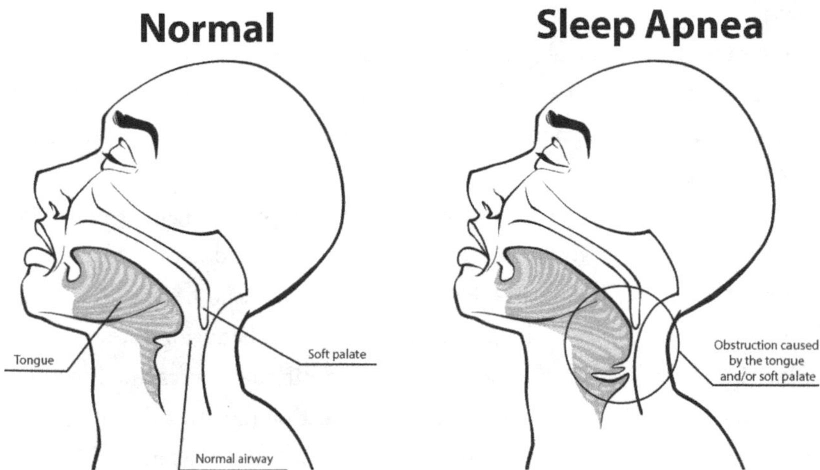

FIGURE 3. Normal versus Obstructed Airway

Central Sleep Apnea

Unlike its more common counterpart *obstructive* sleep apnea, central sleep apnea is not caused by a physical blockage. This type of apnea is indeed *central*, meaning it happens due to the suppression of the respiratory center located in the brain stem.

The central nervous system acts as a command system for many of the body's major functions, including reflexes, memory and learning, control of movement, and regulating internal body temperature. The central nervous system also regulates breathing. When this area of the brain is suppressed, breathing is slower and more prone to interruptions.

Common causes for central sleep apnea are pain medications, sleep aids, and hypnotics that suppress the breathing center. Rarely, brain tumors and brain malformation (Chiari malformation) can also impinge on the breathing center and suppress the respiratory drive.

Central sleep apnea is differentiated from obstructive apnea during a sleep study as there's a visible lack of effort from the chest muscles and diaphragm. That's because there is no signal from the brain cuing these body parts to inhale. This lack of chest movement is recognizable during a sleep study, illustrating the difference between central sleep apnea and obstructive sleep apnea, in which the body is trying quite hard to breathe, but is encountering an obstruction.

Sometimes central sleep apnea can occur when CPAP therapy is introduced, which is called treatment-induced central sleep apnea. This usually resolves with time.

Connor

Connor was a 17-year-old high school student who came to me with complaints of significant daytime fatigue and mild headaches. Connor was so tired that he even fell asleep in the waiting room prior to his appointment time. His mom had also noticed him snoring.

When I examined him, I found Connor to be a typical teenager who loved sports and who would rather be on the soccer field and not at the doctor's office. Despite his fondness for sports, during the past few months, Connor said he was tired most of the time and was upset that he hadn't been able to give 100% during games.

Since his mom wasn't in the room, Connor admitted he occasionally smoked pot, thinking that could improve his sleep, but he wasn't taking any other medications or any hard drugs. He was mildly overweight, and I noticed that he had prominently enlarged tonsils.

An in-lab study is recommended for children 18 or younger, so because of Connor's age, that's what we did. The study revealed mild OSA. On careful review, he also had significant central apneic events, meaning that there was no movement of the chest or abdomen (the lack of effort I mentioned earlier), pointing toward central sleep apnea. In other words, Connor was suffering from both types of sleep apnea: obstructive *and* central.

I discussed Connor's results with him and his mom and strongly recommended that this problem needed to be looked at further. I also got his primary care physician involved, and we proceeded with a magnetic resonance imaging (MRI) of the brain. The MRI revealed Chiari malformation (where portions of the brain bulge through the skull-base opening), compressing the breathing center, resulting in the occurrence of central apneic events.

Connor had his tonsils and adenoids removed, which resolved the obstructive apnea episodes. To treat the central sleep apnea, Connor had a neurosurgical evaluation. He is being watched closely by this neurosurgeon, with serial MRIs conducted to look for any changes so they can intervene surgically, if needed.

How Sleep Apnea Is Diagnosed

I recommend that anyone with symptoms of sleep apnea schedule a consultation with a sleep specialist so that the appropriate testing can be determined. However, many people drag their feet when it comes time to make this appointment. One reason is that they assume the test will be an in-lab sleep study, which they are naturally leery of.

"Who wants to or can sleep in a strange environment?" many of my clients complain. Thankfully, for most people, an at-home sleep study will suffice.

Over the past decade, home sleep testing has become a convenient and cost-effective method for diagnosing sleep apnea. A home testing kit can be picked up at the doctor's office, and the testing can be done at the comfort of your own home. The kit is returned the next day, and the information can be downloaded so that the doctor can interpret the data.

I prefer the WatchPAT® home sleep test device, which is a sophisticated device that monitors any constriction of the arteries (or peripheral arterial tone), as well as oxygen levels, snoring, body position, and sleep stages. Home sleep apnea tests can, however, underestimate the severity of sleep apnea; thus, we cannot rule out sleep apnea even if the test is negative. (In such instances, I refer folks for an in-lab sleep study, the gold standard diagnostic methodology for sleep apnea.)

By analyzing the data from the home test, the physician can then determine the type and severity of the apnea. In my practice, I estimate that 95% of the studies I perform are home-based. There are exceptions to this rule, like when I suspect a person has a complicated sleep disorder diagnosis like narcolepsy, or if they have associated medical conditions like congestive heart failure or emphysema.

In-lab studies, where you spend the night at a sleep center, provide much more detailed information by measuring sleep waves, breathing patterns, limb movements, chin muscle tone, heart rate, eye movements, snoring, awakenings, oxygen saturation, body position, types of apneas, whether the blockage is partial or complete, and more.

If there is suspicion of narcolepsy or hypersomnia (discussed in detail in upcoming chapters), a daytime study is also warranted to assess the severity of daytime drowsiness (somnolence) and fatigue.

Treatment for Sleep Apnea

Before the 1980s, a tracheostomy was the only known treatment for sleep apnea. A tracheotomy is a surgical procedure in which an incision is made in the front of the neck into the windpipe (the trachea) and a tube is inserted. Back then, this was the only way that doctors knew to bypass the obstruction in the throat that causes OSA.[41] Thankfully, today people have many more and far less invasive options!

For most of my apnea patients, the first step is to determine the root cause of their apnea and trying to address it directly. This includes identifying potential treatable causes like weight gain.

Obesity is the leading cause of OSA. Weight is distributed evenly around the body, and when a person is too heavy, fat deposition around the throat causes narrowing of the airways. Even a 10% loss in weight can have a significant impact on sleep apnea treatment.

Although weight loss is strongly recommended, it doesn't always cure apnea.

Other treatable causes include a deviated nasal septum, extra tissue in the back of the throat, and nasal polyps. These problems can all be fixed with routine surgery. By relieving the obstruction that was causing the blockage, the symptoms of mild sleep apnea can be fixed permanently.

Several lifestyle changes can also make a difference. Avoidance of alcohol, which relaxes the muscles of the throat, and stopping smoking, which causes upper airway inflammation, can also help relieve sleep apnea. People who eat earlier in the evening, as opposed to late at night, also fare better.[42]

I also advise that my clients with mild sleep apnea learn to sleep on their sides since side-sleeping is a better position for those diagnosed with sleep apnea. Lying on the back worsens sleep apnea, as gravity causes the tongue to fall backward, obstructing the airway in the back of the throat.

Some of my clients go as far as to place a tennis ball behind them in bed so that they have a physical reminder to avoid rolling onto their backs. This is called positional therapy and is only indicated for patients with mild positional sleep apnea. There are also several devices on the market that administer a small shock if you accidentally roll over to your back while sleeping.

Devices Used in the Treatment of Sleep Apnea

CPAP (continuous positive airway pressure, as you may remember) is well known and the gold standard in the treatment of obstructive sleep apnea. This is a small device with a compressor that blows air through a hose into the nostrils to open the airway.

The CPAP literally acts like a splint to keep the airway open, and the tongue (which is the major cause of obstruction) out of the airway. The machine also has the capacity to adjust humidity. There is a heating element, as well, which keeps the air and tubing warm. Modern CPAP machines also include a feature to ramp up the airway pressure once you've fallen asleep. This avoids blasts of strong air while you are trying to fall sleep. These features are standard these days, making CPAP treatment more tolerable.

Most devices also feature auto-capacity, which adjusts the range of pressure as needed. This has been a major advancement in technology as there is no need for a fixed pressure all the time. This feature has also increased tolerance and compliance for many.

Since CPAP machines are constantly blowing air, some patients have difficulty exhaling. CPAP machines also have settings to help with this, called an expiratory pressure relief feature. But for this feature to be functional, the setting needs to be turned on.

If patients still have difficulty exhaling—especially in patients who have COPD—I prescribe **BiPAP** therapy where there are two pressure settings, one for inhaling (IPAP) and one for exhaling (EPAP). The EPAP pressure is lower than IPAP, which helps with expelling the air.

There is another phenomenon that can result in patients not tolerating CPAP, called treatment-induced central apnea. This occurs when a person responds to air from the CPAP by hyperventilating, thus resulting in low levels of carbon dioxide in your blood. Carbon dioxide is a breathing stimulant, and when this is washed up, the respiratory drive to breathe is suppressed, resulting in treatment-induced central sleep apnea. This usually resolves with time, but if it is persistent or when central sleep apnea is caused by chronic use of narcotics, I use another available methodology called adaptive servo ventilation (ASV). The ASV device adapts to your breathing pattern rather than forcing air and forcing you to breathe in sync with the machine. This uses a more sophisticated algorithm that helps sync with your breathing and must be managed by a sleep specialist or a physician who has expertise in this field.

There are also **different types of masks** to help deliver consistent pressure. In my practice, I use facial contour detection software that helps to custom fit masks for my clients. Introducing more choices in the mask department has helped a lot with tolerance and compliance. There is no need to wear the old Darth Vader-type masks any longer!

Beyond CPAP, folks with sleep apnea have several new choices for managing their condition. The **eXciteOSA**[43] device is a clinically proven, US Food and Drug Administration (FDA) authorized daytime therapy for the treatment of mild OSA or snoring. The device is placed on the tongue for 20 minutes each day for the first six weeks to improve tongue muscle function, thus preventing tongue collapse and obstruction at night. This treatment is repeated twice a week for 20 minutes as maintenance therapy.

As stated earlier, with age, our airway and tongue muscles—particularly the genioglossus—lose tonicity. The device applies low-frequency electrical stimulation to improve the tone of the tongue and upper airway muscles and help prevent airway collapse.[44] The best part is that the treatment can be performed any time during the day or before going to sleep. It eliminates the need for any nighttime treatment, which is why many mild sleep apnea clients are trying it.

Oral appliances—only indicated for mild to moderate sleep apnea—are custom-made by dentists who specialize in sleep apnea treatment. These work by moving the lower jaw forward, thus moving the tongue out of the air passage, and thereby relieving the obstruction.

Once placed, a follow-up sleep study is required to determine the efficacy of the device. One issue with these devices is that by moving the jaw forward they can cause jaw pain, so caution is advised. There are several over-the-counter oral appliances on the market, but they are not as effective as the custom-fit ones.

Surgical Treatment for Sleep Apnea

Throughout the years, physicians have used various surgical options to treat sleep apnea. Unfortunately, many of these were not as effective as physicians hoped, which is why CPAP treatment is still the gold standard for most apnea clients. That said, it's worth getting an overview of surgeries that can also help with snoring.

Uvulopalatopharygoplasty is a surgery to remove extra tissue from the throat to improve the flow of breath. Commonly referred to as Up3, it normally involves removing the uvula, soft palate, and excess tissue at the back of the throat area (the posterior pharynx). Up3 was popular in the late 90s but has since fallen by the wayside as it is not as effective in controlling the collapse of the remaining soft tissue as once thought. The pain and discomfort associated with this procedure were also significant drawbacks that caused Up3 to fall out of favor.

Somnoplasty is a similar but less invasive procedure that uses a laser, rather than physical cutting, to reduce the soft tissue in the upper airway. This procedure has been shown to reduce snoring, but it is not as effective at treating sleep apnea.

Pillar implants is another surgical option that has mostly lost popularity. In this procedure, surgeons implant pillars into the roof of the mouth to help prevent collapse. This has not been very useful as the tongue is the major contributor to the obstruction.

Mandibular advancement surgery is another type of surgery sometimes used to treat sleep apnea. It is a surgical correction of the lower jaw, mainly to advance it forward to relieve the obstruction. Sometimes, this mandibular advancement surgery is also combined with the correction of other jaw abnormalities. This procedure is performed by oral and maxillary surgeons who are experts in this type of surgery.

For folks with a deviated nasal septum, **nasal surgery** may provide some relief by correcting any asymmetry, thereby relieving obstructions.

For children who are diagnosed with sleep apnea, having a **tonsillectomy** or **adenoidectomy** provides relief by removing airway obstruction caused by the tonsils and adenoids.

Inspire® therapy is another option that recently came on the market, and it's being marketed as an alternative sleep apnea treatment for those who can't tolerate a CPAP machine. It is a hypoglossal nerve stimulator reserved for people with moderate to severe sleep apnea.

With this type of therapy, a pulse generator is surgically placed inside the chest wall cavity, and the stimulator lead is placed on the hypoglossal nerve that serves the tongue. With every breath, a minimal electric impulse stimulates the tongue to protrude forward, thus preventing the closure of the upper airway. You turn the device on and off with a remote control, but there's a lag time so stimulation only starts once you've fallen asleep.

Though this option is invasive, I have several clients who are doing well with Inspire therapy. The procedure seems to have resolved their sleep apnea, and they are happy that they do not need to deal with CPAP masks and hoses.

Medications for Sleep Apnea

Modafinil, armodafinil, and solriamfetol are FDA-approved medications used to treat residual daytime sleepiness related to sleep apnea. There are also newer medications on the horizon for the treatment of sleep apnea. Research is underway to combine medications like oxybutynin and atomoxetine, which can help reduce airway collapse.

Over-the-Counter Treatments for Sleep Apnea

In addition to these doctor-prescribed options, there are several over-the-counter remedies for sleep apnea. These include nasal strips, oral devices, throat sprays, and more. While people may find some brief relief from these, they never solve the problem 100%. Most of them improve snoring without addressing the underlying cause of sleep apnea.

Several mattress and pillow companies have also started to advertise their products as solutions to sleep apnea. These products can help minimally, especially the cooling and pressure-relieving mattress options. The cold environment does help the secretion of melatonin, and the pressure-relieving types may even relieve pain by adjusting the spine and neck and can help to sleep better. However, they cannot fix the airway obstruction that is the major contributor to the problem.

People are spending thousands of dollars on such beds, and most will claim they sleep better, reflecting the desire to solve the problem from the outside in while the solution to relieve the obstruction needs to be from the inside out.

So, if you, your spouse, or your children snore, or you notice them stopping breathing during the night, please call your health care provider immediately. Untreated sleep apnea can result in harmful effects, affecting various organs, cognitive function, mental health, and, as seen in Sam's case, it can even result in death. For that reason, *being proactive about your sleep health truly is a matter of life and death.*

Many people avoid getting evaluated because they're scared of being diagnosed with sleep apnea. However, once the diagnosis is made and you receive treatment, you will have more energy, a happier mood, and better overall health.

CPAP Intolerance

Liz walked into my office carrying a big, brown box. She looked very frustrated. Liz was a 28-year-old kindergarten teacher who moved from Alaska to teach at a school near my office and had come to see me for a second opinion as she was not tolerating her CPAP.

Liz had been diagnosed with severe sleep apnea and was prescribed CPAP therapy. She said she "tried using this contraption" for three months and was ready to "throw it out the window." According to Liz, the pressure was too much, and she felt bloated. To make matters worse, the mask was causing irritation on her nose and lips.

Though Liz had tried different masks, she was frustrated and had given up using the CPAP. But recently her blood pressure had shot up and she almost had an accident when she started to fall asleep at the wheel on her way to school one morning. She knew she really needed to get things figured out and was desperate for help.

After examining her, my sense was that things had not been set up right. Her machine was working fine and was set at a fixed pressure of 13, meaning it blows a set pressure of 13 cmH2O all the time. Adjusting a CPAP machine is an easy fix, and most modern CPAPs have an auto-adjusting capacity and can use variable pressure to keep the airway open.

I set Liz on a range of 8–14 cmH2O. Next, I used a facial recognition app to provide a better fitted mask, as hers was causing pressure points at the bridge of her nose and around her lips, causing irritation and skin breakdown.

When Liz came in for a follow-up visit a few months later, she reported she had finally gotten used to her CPAP. Best of all, her blood pressure was well controlled.

She was happy to report that this had a positive effect on her class as she was feeling so much happier.

☽

Here's the thing: ***If you don't use your CPAP machine, it won't help.*** And unfortunately, many people aren't using their CPAP machines as prescribed. As many as 50% of people don't use their CPAP machine as directed by their physician, meaning they only use it occasionally, only wear it part of the night, or simply stop using it all together after a while. Sadly, these folks won't receive the benefits of boosted energy and protection against cognitive decline.

One of the main reasons for not tolerating CPAP is issues with the mask or finding the right pressure, but as I mentioned, those are easy to fix.

If you're having a hard time tolerating CPAP therapy, talk to your doctor about potential pressure adjustments or consider other treatment options that are now available.

Hypersomnia: Sleeping Too Much

Idiopathic hypersomnia (IH) and narcolepsy (discussed later in this chapter) are extremely debilitating conditions, as you'll see in Ashley and Logan's stories. These are often misdiagnosed as depression, sleep apnea, or even laziness.

The reason why folks with these conditions appear depressed is that they are tired from not getting the rest they require, and they often have brain fog. They often see multiple specialists (psychiatrists, nutritionists, psychologists, and neurologists) before someone suggests that the issue could be sleep-related. The time to diagnose IH and narcolepsy is typically between 7 and 10 years.

Ashley

Ashley was a 38-year-old woman who worked at a social media marketing firm. Her manager had recently written her up, and she was on the verge of losing her job. She was taking a lot of time off work, using her paid time off for self-care, but was still noticeably tired and withdrawn.

A concerned friend and coworker had noticed Ashley falling asleep during meetings and made her promise that she would see a sleep specialist.

Ashley told me she had been having these issues since she was 16, and that she had tried everything—multivitamins, caffeine pills, energy drinks, and even stimulant pills from friends who she knew had access to these medications (she said she didn't ask too many questions).

She mentioned she sleeps about 10–12 hours each night. Still feeling tired, Ashley has tried to sleep *longer*, but it didn't help. She napped regularly, but that too, wasn't helpful. She even had an MRI of her brain, and there were no abnormalities.

Ashley hadn't had any head trauma or viral illnesses. She went to see a psychiatrist who diagnosed her with depression due to the excessive daytime fatigue. She started on antidepressants, which didn't help. In fact, she felt worse at times.

She said her college years were a struggle as she couldn't stay up late and was often made fun of for being a "party pooper." Ashley said she basically survived those years on lots of coffee, energy drinks, and even got a prescription for stimulants like Adderall from her primary care doctor.

She got an office job in 2019, and she was barely surviving. When the pandemic hit in 2020, Ashley was relieved to work from home where she could take several naps, and while she slept longer hours, she relied on coffee and energy drinks to get her through the day.

When she had to return to the office in 2022, her trouble with staying awake became obvious, and she was on the verge of losing her job.

We did blood work, which came back normal, and her urinalysis showed she was free of any sedatives or illicit drugs. Next, I asked her to keep a detailed Sleep Journal and complete the Sleep Assessment, and I scheduled an in-lab sleep study and a nap study for the following day.

The sleep study did not reveal evidence of other sleep disorders—she was breathing well and sleeping deeply. However, the nap study showed severe sleepiness with an average sleep onset time of seven minutes. She fell asleep on all five naps. Ashley did not, however, go into REM sleep during those naps.

Ashley ultimately ended up with a diagnosis of IH—excessive sleepiness without obvious treatable causes. I was able to discuss the results with her and start her on a stimulant medication called modafinil.

After a month on modafinil and keeping good sleep hygiene, Ashley felt significantly better and was more productive and energetic at work. Her friend who had referred her to me told her she seemed much happier and "with it."

As for Ashley, she said, "It was like my whole world has turned around." She was more cheerful and was able to discontinue the antidepressants as she had a stimulant deficiency rather than depression.

By treating the primary cause, we found a long-term solution to the problem rather than a Band-Aid that only treats the symptoms. Ashley may be on modafinil indefinitely, but for a severe case like hers, it's necessary for her work and quality of life.

Idiopathic Hypersomnia

Being tired is a hallmark of modern-day life. Most of us wish we had fewer responsibilities and more time to rest. However, for folks suffering from hypersomnia, feeling exhausted is just their daily modus operandi, regardless of how much sleep they get. They feel a desperate need for more sleep, even if they're in a calm stage of life and are getting plenty of rest at night.

Hypersomnia simply means sleeping too much and being tired despite getting at least eight hours of sleep each night.

This is different from simply racking up a sleep debt from a busy weekend. In people with hypersomnia, sleepiness persists despite arranging their schedule to get more sleep. They have trouble pulling themselves out of bed in the morning and after naps. When they do get up, they often feel drowsy and irritable throughout the day, longing to collapse back onto their pillow. Often, people with hypersomnia struggle to be productive at work or at school because of their overwhelming fatigue.

As the *idiopathic* in the name suggests, there is no known cause for hypersomnia. This can make it a tricky disorder to diagnose. Because the symptoms—extreme tiredness, an irresistible urge to sleep, and poor concentration—resemble those of many other disorders, diagnosing hypersomnia requires a thorough investigation.

Despite how common the symptoms are, this syndrome seems to be unique to each person, and therefore, a customized treatment plan is usually required.

What Causes IH?

The exact cause of this disorder is still unknown. While there may not be one known root cause for IH, scientists are aware of several influencing factors. For one thing, people with hypersomnia seem to have lower levels of histamine, serotonin, and acetylcholine, stimulants that keep us awake and alert during the day. There also seem to be irregularities involving two types of neurochemicals: hypocretins and prostaglandin D2 (or PGD2).

There are two types of hypocretins—hypocretin-1 and hypocretin-2 (now called orexin-1 and orexin-2)—and they both promote wakefulness and muscle tone.

Prostaglandin D2, on the other hand, is a known somnogen, a neurochemical that promotes sleepiness and is present in people both with *and* without hypersomnia. In those *without* hypersomnia, PGD2 is counterbalanced by adenosine, a wakefulness-promoting chemical in the brain.

Scientists believe that people with hypersomnia have an overabundance of PGD2 and not enough adenosine to balance it, making it hard for them to stay awake. While they don't understand exactly how these neurochemicals contribute to hypersomnia, they know that they do play a significant role.

Beyond these chemical imbalances, IH can occur due to some medical conditions, medications, or lifestyle choices—including the use or overuse of opiates, hypnotics/sedatives, anti-epileptics, and antipsychotics.

Secondary hypersomnia can occur when a person has had a head injury, stroke, or a neurogenerative, psychiatric, or genetic disorder.

Narcolepsy: Falling Asleep Anytime, Anywhere

Logan was a 19-year-old high school senior who was excited about going to college on a gymnastic scholarship. However, at a recent gymnastics practice, he was found sound asleep in the gym, and it was difficult to wake him up. The school and his parents were all concerned, and they wanted him to be evaluated as soon as possible as he would be going off to college soon.

Logan had already been evaluated by a psychologist and a psychiatrist. He had been treated briefly for depression, but that didn't provide any relief. In fact, the medications made him feel even more groggy, only compounding the problem.

He had also been evaluated by a neurologist who found no neurological abnormality. This specialist happened to be my friend, and he recognized that this could be a sleep issue. So, he referred Logan to me.

Logan came to my office accompanied by his mom, Emily. He told me that ever since middle school, he was always tired. He said he was always fighting the tiredness, but nothing seemed to help. He was often made fun of and called "sleepy head," and he'd often go off by himself rather than hang out with his friends.

During the evaluation, I used the Epworth sleepiness scale to measure Logan's level of sleepiness. Anything above 10 is considered concerning. Logan scored 18.

Logan also mentioned that when something exciting happens—like after he sticks his landing on a vault or wins a competition—he feels like his face droops a bit. He also feels weak in his knees during these moments.

Logan reported that he doesn't sleep well at night and typically wakes up several times, but he figured this was probably stress since he was a senior and there was lots going on. He also confessed that there were a few instances when he couldn't get up in the mornings because he felt paralyzed. He said that it was extremely frightening and had no idea why it happened.

The first time he mentioned this to his mother, she told him it was probably just a nightmare. But he told me it happened a few other times, and he managed to stay quiet and calm his nerves. He didn't discuss his further paralysis episodes with his family, as he didn't want to burden them with concern.

When I asked about his extended family, Logan mentioned he had heard stories that his late great uncle was known to fall sound asleep at church and at family gatherings. He had heard that the uncle had been diagnosed with a sleep disorder, but Logan didn't know much about it.

As a sleep specialist, it was clear to me that Logan had the classic signs and symptoms of narcolepsy. In fact, facial drooping was a bit of a giveaway as it is caused by a sudden onset of REM sleep that knocks out the facial muscles. (This kind of facial drooping is not the same as we'd see when a person has a stroke or in someone with Bell's palsy, when the nerve completely stops working.)

Clinically, the symptoms of facial drooping and feeling weak at his knees are consistent with cataplexy, the sudden weakness or loss of muscle control.[45] Cataplexy can be triggered by strong feelings like surprise, laughter, stress, excitement, or fear. This is the key feature in the diagnosis of narcolepsy. The cataplexy can be subtle, as in Logan's case, but it can also be as dramatic as collapsing while remaining fully conscious.

Logan had an overnight in-lab study, which didn't reveal any significant sleep disorders, but he had four REM sleep episodes on his nap study with a mean sleep latency (time to go to sleep) of four minutes. This is the classic finding in narcolepsy.

I treated Logan with two medications: sodium oxybate and solriamfetol. This provided dramatic improvement in his symptoms. After a follow-up visit, we tapered him off solriamfetol, and now that Logan's in college, he continues to do well.

Even though he has some days when he feels tired—like many college students do—most days are great, and Logan's overall quality of life has significantly improved. He continues to compete in gymnastics without any cataplexy, and as his grades show, he's thriving academically.

It's too bad he didn't get help earlier, but today, Logan is doing well. He is stable and no longer battling fatigue every waking minute of the day.

In the 2001 film *Rat Race*, Rowan Atkinson portrayed a narcoleptic who would frequently fall into unexpected, standing naps at the drop of a hat. In the movie, narcolepsy was used as a comedic effect. However, folks with this condition may not find these depictions amusing.

For one thing, narcolepsy can seriously affect quality of life. Folks with narcolepsy may have poor sleep quality and poor academic performance. They may also have difficulty driving, holding down a job, and navigating social situations due to their inability to stay awake.

In addition, media portrayals of narcolepsy often confuse napping with symptoms of cataplexy. A nap, of course, is a short sleep during the day, while cataplexy is the sudden, uncontrollable loss of muscle control brought on by strong emotions.[46]

Narcolepsy is a sleep and neurological syndrome that is primarily caused by the deficiency of awake-producing chemicals in the brain. Narcolepsy often runs in families, and it is a disabling disorder with significant emotional and physical components.

The daytime sleepiness can be quite profound, affecting the day-to-day functioning. Folks with narcolepsy also complain of poor sleep at night. Most people cannot function in real life without appropriate treatment.

The lack of wakefulness chemicals in those with narcolepsy is due to the destruction of hypocretins, also known as orexin. These cells control a wide range of outputs related to our awakening and motivated behaviors.[47] They are located in the portion of the brain called the hypothalamus, which is responsible for regulating sleep, appetite, and temperature. The cells also promote the secretion of stimulating neurotransmitters like histamine, serotonin, dopamine, norepinephrine, and acetylcholine.

More than 90% of hypocretin cells are missing in narcoleptics.[48] The exact cause is unknown, but narcolepsy is believed to be related to an autoimmune process that mistakes hypocretins as enemies and destroys them.

Genetic and environmental factors are believed to contribute to narcolepsy, although scientists have not pinpointed an exact genome that is responsible for the syndrome.

Discovery of Narcolepsy

Narcolepsy was first described in medical literature in 1880 by French physician Jean-Baptist Gélineau, the first doctor to connect all the symptoms of narcolepsy and group them under one diagnosis.

The word narcolepsy comes from two Greek words: *narke*, meaning numbness and *lepsis*, meaning attack. Dr. Gélineau first began treating his patients with bromide and arsenic, which showed some effectiveness in his more severe patients.[49] Fortunately, there are much better medications available today to treat narcolepsy.

The incidence of narcolepsy is roughly one in 2,000 people in the general population, but this disorder is significantly underdiagnosed. The presenting symptoms often show up during teenage years, although they can be diagnosed as late as in the 30s.[50]

Classic Symptoms of Narcolepsy

These symptoms are often indicators of narcolepsy:

- **Sleepiness and fatigue.** People often have significant and debilitating fatigue during the day. This is mainly due to the poor quality of sleep the night before. The exhaustion is persistent and cannot be resolved with improving sleep routines or sleeping longer.
- **Cataplexy.** Sudden muscle weakness and loss of tone causing one to collapse but with preserved consciousness. This is triggered by strong emotions. It can be subtle—like the buckling of knees, drooping of eye lids, nodding of the head—or a dramatic collapse, like a sack of potatoes. Most people have mild and nonspecific symptoms and are able to wade through these spells.
- **Sleep paralysis.** People with narcolepsy may suffer from a sudden, scary inability to move their limbs or head when they first wake up. It only lasts a few seconds, and it often can occur when a person is waking up or drifting off to sleep. While occasional episodes can happen after sleep deprivation, the phenomenon occurs more frequently in narcoleptics.
- **Poor sleep quality.** Most folks with narcolepsy have poor sleep quality and wake up multiple times at night. They never feel rested when they wake up.

These classic symptoms must all be present to diagnose narcolepsy. However, some people may also experience additional symptoms like hallucinations and vivid dreams. These dreams and hallucinations are often frightening, and they can happen at any time during the night. The hallucinations that happen immediately before you've completely fallen asleep are called hypnagogic. When they occur while you're waking up, are called hypnopompic.

Another non-classic symptom is automatic behaviors, which include sudden sleep attacks where people continue with what they are doing, like writing, typing, or driving while they're asleep, and when they awaken, they are confused and do not have any recollection of falling asleep.

Types of Narcolepsy

Narcolepsy is divided into type 1 and type 2. Type 1 narcoleptic patients often present with symptoms of cataplexy (the sudden, uncontrollable loss of muscle control brought on by strong emotions, as you may recall).

Sleep studies show that narcoleptics enter REM sleep very early in the sleep cycle. In type 1 narcolepsy, REM sleep can also occur when a person is *awake* and cause cataplexy.

In type 2 narcolepsy, the classic symptoms may or may not be apparent, and they lack symptoms of cataplexy.

Diagnosing Hypersomnia and Narcolepsy

The symptoms of excessive daytime drowsiness should have persisted at least three months before a person is evaluated for these conditions. The person must also be allowed enough time for sleep, not simply going to bed too late and not sleeping enough, as that's a different issue.

It's important in the initial consultation for your doctor to get a detailed history and lab work to make sure there are no other sleep disorders or other medical conditions like thyroid hormone deficiency or anemia.

There are also prescription medications that may have a sedative effect on the person. A Sleep Journal and actigraphy—wearing a device on the wrist to measure movement—can help investigate one's sleep pattern, making sure they sleep sufficiently and identify any poor sleep routines and practices.

Next, an overnight in-lab sleep study can rule out other sleep disorders. In these cases, an in-lab study is required since home studies cannot document some of the details like the quality of sleep, onset of REM sleep, limb movements, and any episodes of partial or complete interruption of breathing. These details are needed to rule out sleep apnea, limb movement, or other sleep disorders.

The in-lab sleep test is followed the next morning with multiple sleep latency testing, a series of five nap opportunities to assess the severity of sleepiness and detect onset of REM sleep, if any. The nap study lasts for 20 minutes, and we typically perform five in a row. We take the mean number of minutes that it took the person to fall asleep over all five nap tests. If they fall asleep in eight minutes or less, on average, they are probably experiencing hypersomnia.

Also, REM sleep should never occur during the day. If the average mean sleep onset is eight minutes or less and there is one or no REM periods, then this is consistent with the diagnosis of IH.

If there are two or more REM sleep episodes during a nap test, and if the average time to fall asleep is less than eight minutes, it points to a diagnosis of narcolepsy.

Another practical clue from clinical history is that naps are refreshing in patients with narcolepsy but not so for those with hypersomnia.

There are also blood tests measuring human leukocyte antigen genotypes that show some association to narcolepsy, but these tests are not conclusive. When the diagnosis of narcolepsy is entertained, an MRI of the brain may also be needed in some cases to rule out any brain lesions.

The gold standard for diagnosing narcolepsy is to measure hypocretin in the cerebrospinal fluid. This is achieved by doing a lumbar puncture (a spinal tap). Normally the levels are greater than 200 pg/ml. If the value of hypocretin-1 in the spinal fluid is less than 110 pg/ml, it is highly suggestive of narcolepsy. (Very few labs specialize in measuring this.)

Because this procedure is invasive, I typically only use it as a last resort if there are diagnostic challenges. In my 25 years of practice, I've only ordered this test twice to confirm the diagnosis.

Treatment for Idiopathic Hypersomnia

The most effective treatment for IH is good sleep habits, sufficient sleep time, and structure. The cornerstone of treatment for this condition is stimulant medications like methylphenidate, amphetamines, and wake-promoting medications like modafinil and armodafinil. There has also been recent FDA approval for sodium oxybate for the treatment of this condition.[51]

Treatments for Narcolepsy

Narcolepsy has no definite cure. Understanding the disease process and enlisting the support of family, friends, and employers can help tremendously in dealing with the unique challenges faced. There are also several effective treatments that can help manage the condition.

Treatment starts with adequate sleep of 8–10 hours. To combat daytime sleepiness, options include stimulants like methylphenidate, amphetamine, modafinil, armodafinil, and solriamfetol. Unfortunately, these stimulant medications do not improve nighttime symptoms or cataplexy. And they can sometimes have side effects like increased heart rate, increased blood pressure, anxiety, insomnia, irritability, and nervousness, so they must be carefully monitored.

Thankfully, drugs like sodium oxybate and the newer compound of sodium oxybate with less sodium are available. The exact mechanism is still not completely understood, but it is a GABA derivative, which helps narcolepsy patients get more and deeper sleep at night. By restoring sleep efficiency and sleep architecture at night, it reduces extreme sleepiness during the day. These are highly controlled medications that need to be prescribed by experts in this field.

There is another newer medicine available called pitolisant that promotes wakefulness by increasing histamines in the brain. (As you may know, histamines keep you awake, and antihistamines put you to sleep.)

SSRIs (selective serotonin reuptake inhibitors) and other antidepressants like fluoxetine, venlafaxine, and tricyclic antidepressants like imipramine and protriptyline have been tried to treat cataplexy. However, they were not very effective and are no longer used. Sodium oxybate and pitolisant are especially helpful if folks are suffering from cataplexy.

In addition to medications, improving sleep routines is mandatory. Maintaining a strict sleep schedule with at least eight hours of sleep is highly recommended, as is avoiding gaining excess weight. Naps are often refreshing for narcoleptics, and I have even prescribed scheduled naps at work and school for my patients with narcolepsy.

There is research that suggests identifying the autoimmune response that destroys orexin-producing cells and using medications like steroids and intravenous immunoglobulin therapy to stop that process may be helpful. (Immunoglobulin is a protein that helps the body fight infection.)

Plasmapheresis (a process by which a machine separates the red and white blood cells, platelets, and plasma) may also help stop the autoimmune process. Other promising treatments are being tested. These include implanting orexin cells, gene therapy to help the expression of hypocretins, and administering orexin through the nose or intravenously.

Prognosis

The symptoms of IH and narcolepsy ebb and flow. Fortunately, with newer medications and support from family, school and at the workplace, patients with these conditions can lead a near normal life. It's my hope that with better education, patients won't have to wait so long for a diagnosis in the future.

Other Sleep Disorders

By this point, you may feel like an expert in sleep disorders. Though I've covered the most common sleep problems, I've yet to explore some of the less-talked-about forms of sleep disorders.

While the following tend to affect fewer folks, they can still be difficult to manage for those who experience them. It's worth learning a little about each one so you can recognize the signs and symptoms.

Tracy

Tracy was a 55-year-old weary looking woman who came to my office. When I invited her to sit, she all but collapsed into the chair and wept.

She told me she had a history of sleep apnea, and she was faithfully using her CPAP machine every night. Recently, she was experiencing a crawly sensation and an urge to move her legs, especially in the evening. She also had an aching sensation in her legs.

Most nights, Tracy and her family would relax in their family room and watch a show or movie. But Tracy said she just couldn't sit still. She *had* to pace around. Because she had to be constantly on the move to get relief for her symptoms, her family was concerned for her, and she was upset that she couldn't spend quality time with them in the evenings because her fidgeting and pacing disturbed everyone.

She had tried various over-the-counter medications like magnesium and vitamins without much relief and had seen her family doctor about the issue (who really didn't know what to do). That's when she was referred to me.

It was totally understandable that Tracy was in tears. She was desperate to get help for her condition.

I ordered blood work, and it showed she had significant iron deficiency, so I prescribed an iron supplement. Most people get relief when their iron levels are corrected, but Tracy continued to have persistent symptoms. Next, I prescribed pramipexole, which helped significantly.

Tracy had some side effects from the medication—drowsiness and mild nausea—during the daytime, so I lowered her dosage. When she still had some residual symptoms, I added gabapentin. This combination resolved her problems.

During her follow-up visit, Tracy was doing well, her symptoms were under control, and she was able to snuggle on the couch with her husband and kids again and watch TV with them.

Restless Leg Syndrome and Periodic Limb Movement Disorder

Restless leg syndrome (RLS)—what Tracy had—is a condition in which people report the uncomfortable and irresistible urge to move their legs, most commonly in the evenings.

This is a powerful sensation where the person is driven to try and alleviate the feelings through movement to try and get the muscles to calm down. It is more than just trying to get settled and comfortable.

Originally called Ekbom disease, this condition typically improves when the person is able to get up and walk around. When the person is still, such as if they're sitting in a classroom or on a plane, the sensation usually intensifies.

Even though this syndrome has existed for centuries, there is minimal awareness about RLS in the public.

If the symptoms associated with RLS occur during sleep and you also experience limb movements, it may be a sign of periodic limb movement disorder. PLMD can be debilitating as it causes frequent awakenings that result in significant daytime sleepiness.

What causes RLS and PLMD? The most common cause for RLS is simply an iron deficiency. Typically, bloodwork should be done to check the person's iron levels, its precursor ferritin, as well as several other vitamins that play a role in regulating movement. These include vitamin B12, magnesium, and folate.

RLS tends to run in families, and certain races are also more predisposed to this condition.

A 2013 study found RLS is prevalent in 0.1 % of Hispanics, 0.5% of Caucasians, 0.4% of African Americans, and 0.7% of others. The prevalence also varied by countries, with 4.9% in Spain, 8.6% in the UK and 7.6 % in the US.[52] And more than 70% of patients with RLS can also have PLMD.

Several antidepressants like venlafaxine, sertraline, fluoxetine, amitriptyline, and antihistamines can exacerbate PLMD.

Treatment for RLS and PLMD. In adults, if iron levels are low—especially if the ferritin is less than 75 micrograms/dl—then iron replacement is indicated. The enzyme that is responsible for making dopamine (the chemical in the brain that controls movements) is iron-dependent.

If treatment with iron does not help, there are medications like ropinirole, pramipexole and a rotigotine patch that are dopamine agonists. Dosing adjustment should be administered carefully by an expert in this field. If prescribed too liberally, these medications are known to worsen the symptoms, causing restlessness to spread to the upper extremities and sometimes causing symptoms to occur during the day.

A word of caution: These dopamine-agonist medications have common side effects like dry mouth, headaches, and nausea, but compulsory behaviors like gambling are also known to occur. Also, narcotic medications like opiates are highly effective in treating RLS. Due to their side effects and dependence concerns, though, I use these only when I have exhausted other medications and resources.

Beyond medication, exercise and relaxation techniques help to soothe irritated muscles. It's also important to check medications that you are taking, as RLS can be a side effect of certain antihistamines like diphenhydramine and anti-nausea medicines like metoclopramide. Most antidepressants are also known to exacerbate RLS.

There are also several devices on the market targeting RLS. These are either placed under the feet or strapped onto the legs, and they provide a vibrating movement to counterbalance the restless feeling.

For PLMD, the treatment is similar to the treatment regimen for RLS. Also, changing antidepressants will help.

When it comes to testing, sleep studies are rarely needed, except in rare situations when symptoms are worse during sleep (which often point to PLMD), or if other sleep disorders are suspected.

REM Behavior Disorder

REM behavior disorder (RBD) falls under the classification of parasomnia, that is, abnormal activity in sleep. This means that unlike other disorders, people can fall asleep. The problem is what happens *while* they are sleeping.

We enter sleep through non-REM sleep, and roughly 90 minutes later, we enter REM sleep. What happens during REM sleep is dramatically different from what happens during the non-REM stages. As you may recall, REM sleep accounts for 20–25% of our total sleep, and the bulk of it occurs toward the morning hours. Muscles are temporarily paralyzed, breathing is irregular, blood pressure rises, and the eyes move rapidly, hence the name—*rapid eye movement* sleep.

In REM sleep, when dreaming occurs, your muscles are paralyzed to ensure that your body doesn't try to enact whatever scenario your mind is playing out during the dream. Even if you're dreaming that you are running through a forest or jumping rope on a playground, your body should be still.

With RBD (first identified in 1986 by Dr. Schenck and colleagues,[53]), the brain fails to restrain the body's movements, and you end up physically enacting your dreams. This can vary from muscle twitches to talking or pushing, even grabbing or kicking your spouse.

If left untreated, RBD can result in significant injuries to a bed partner and to yourself. Fortunately, the incidence of RBD is less than 1% among adults.

Tom

Tom was a well-built, 58-year-old retired Army Ranger who was brought to the clinic by his wife, Kelly, as Tom had been waking up screaming. During one of his nighttime episodes, he had punched Kelly in his sleep. Tom did not have much recollection of the event, but Kelly certainly did.

Similar episodes had been happening once a year, but recently, they had started to occur more often. Tom had a history of PTSD—post-traumatic stress disorder—for which he had received treatment.

Kelly stated that, aside from a little snoring, Tom usually slept soundly—except for the times when he flails around in his sleep with no recollection of it the next day. This usually happened toward the morning hours.

Kelly could not pinpoint any triggers, but she did mention that one episode had occurred on New Year's Eve after Tom had been drinking excessively and went to bed late. Because these occurrences were becoming more and more frequent, Kelly was concerned that Tom might accidentally hurt her or himself.

This is a typical history for RBD. I sent Tom for an in-lab study. Due to the fact he was snoring, I had to rule out sleep apnea. I also wanted to monitor his limb movements since home sleep studies cannot monitor those.

The sleep study revealed Tom had two episodes that night with sudden and rapid movement, with screaming, and he almost fell off the bed. Fortunately, the technician was on the lookout and restrained him in time. This happened while he was in REM sleep.

The study also revealed he had moderate sleep apnea, and I started him on CPAP therapy. I also added a benzodiazepine medication called clonazepam. Fortunately, that did the trick, and Tom hasn't had any further episodes, even years later.

Men 50 years and older comprise 90% of all the reported cases of RBD. This syndrome can be associated with—or a precursor to—other neurological conditions like Parkinson's disease or Lewy body dementia, which is a form of dementia where protein deposits accumulate in the brain.

In a study published in the *Lancet Neurology* journal in 2006, the incidence of progression to such disorders was as high as 45% when participants were followed for a period of 11.5 years.[54]

Once other sleep disorders like sleep apnea and PLMD have been ruled out, the treatment for RBD usually involves clonazepam. This medication acts by increasing non-REM stage 2 sleep, and as a result, there is less time spent in REM sleep, thereby lowering the chances of these episodes. While clonazepam is effective, we need to be careful about the side effects of this medication. These can include being sleepy the next day, dizziness, and worsening of other sleep disorders like sleep apnea. Plus, it can be addictive.

If this medication is not tolerated, the other option is to use melatonin. Getting an adequate amount of sleep and practicing good sleep hygiene also help people achieve long-term success.

Beyond medication, it's important to create a safe environment in the bedroom by removing objects around the bed so that if an RBD episode occurs, the person won't harm themselves or others. I also recommend the person add soft padding around the bed and furniture and lower their bed level to prevent falling from height.

Sleep-Related Eating Disorder and Nocturnal Eating Syndrome

Maddie was a 67-year-old woman with history of high blood pressure and insomnia. By the time she came to see me, she had been taking zolpidem for two years to help her fall asleep.

Her husband brought her to the office after he noticed that she had been missing from their bedroom in the middle of the night, around 2 a.m. When he got up to look for her, she was in the kitchen eating. When he tried to talk to her, she seemed half-asleep, and he had to escort her back to the bedroom.

It had been a puzzle to him because many mornings there would be open food cans and food crumbs in the kitchen, but Maddie had no recollection of going into the kitchen at night. Meanwhile, she had been steadily gaining weight over the past year.

I recognized her condition as sleep-related eating disorder caused by her sleep aid. Gradually, I was able to wean her off zolpidem and substitute it with another class of medication.

This is a classic example of sleep-related eating disorder (SRED), a condition in which folks eat in their sleep without their knowledge. SRED is classified as a type of parasomnia, an abnormal behavior that occurs during sleep.

People with SRED tend to gain weight without understanding why as they don't have any memory of eating during the night. SRED could be a side effect of medications that are used to treat insomnia, like zolpidem, as well as some antidepressants and anti-psychotic medications. These episodes usually stop when the medication is stopped.

Other causes, like sleep deprivation and primary sleep disorders such as sleep apnea and RLS need to be ruled out before the diagnosis can be established as these disorders can coexist and make SRED worse.

SRED can be dangerous if people attempt to cook food while in a semi-lucid state or if they eat substances that aren't, in fact, food. As far as the treatment for SRED goes, I advise stress management and practicing my *7 Proven Sleep Strategies*, which I recommend to all my clients. I also recommend reassessing the need of sleeping pills. If they do still require sleeping pills, I usually switch to a medication that is less likely to cause SRED.

In nocturnal eating syndrome (NES), on the other hand, people are awake when they eat. They already have insomnia and believe that getting up to eat is the only thing that will help them fall back asleep. For some people, this can happen multiple times a night.

Treatment for SRED and NES usually involves cognitive behavioral therapy, antidepressants, and relaxation exercises that promote sleep. Often patients with these disorders also suffer from associated psychiatric disorders like anxiety and depression. Psychoactive medications they take to manage their conditions may be causing their eating disorder. Thus, managing these disorders could be difficult.

Teeth Grinding

Teeth grinding (or bruxism) is simply the grinding of teeth during sleep. This problem is especially common among clients with sleep apnea. For those folks, the grinding can become so severe that it's audible.

Some people experience teeth grinding because of stress and anxiety rather than sleep apnea. If left untreated, bruxism can cause jaw soreness and tooth damage over time. If sleep apnea is the problem, CPAP or an oral appliance can help. If the grinding is caused by stress, a mouth guard in combination with stress management techniques usually solves the problem.

Jet Lag

Many of us have experienced jet lag at some point in our lives as a result of air travel. Jet lag is simply the inability for your internal clock to adapt to the local time. It is stuck at the place where you were before traveling. The larger the time difference between your place of origin and destination, the worse the jet lag is.

Let's say you depart Los Angeles at 3 p.m. for Frankfurt, Germany. It's an 11-hour flight and a nine-hour time difference, so when you land it's 11 a.m. in Frankfurt, but it's only 2 a.m. in LA where your internal clock is stuck. Your body longs for deep sleep, but you are expected to be awake, whether for a business meeting or to explore. This schedule is worse on the body with eastward travel like the LA to Frankfurt trip as you're losing time and forced to have a shorter sleep cycle.

The brain's SCN (the suprachiasmatic nucleus, as you may recall)—your internal clock—tries its best to help you adjust to your new time zone by taking cues from the light and the surroundings. The drawback is that the SCN is slow to adjust and can only make a one-hour adjustment per 24 hours.

With a nine-hour time difference between LA and Frankfurt during daylight saving time, it means it would take you *nine days* to adapt to the change in time zones. Often, a trip such as this doesn't last nine days, so when you head back to LA, it throws your internal clock into chaos.

Fortunately, jet lag is not as bad traveling westward (Frankfurt to LA) as you gain time (nine hours in this example) and have the luxury to sleep longer.

Jet lag is a major challenge for frequent flyers, pilots, and flight crews. One way to combat this is to take melatonin at around 7 p.m. at the time of your destination. This tricks the brain into thinking it's nighttime. This helps alleviate the clock discrepancy. To lessen the symptoms, I recommend avoiding taking naps upon arrival and keeping up with the time at your destination. Use of caffeine during the day is also helpful to combat sleepiness.

Another strategy involves going to bed an hour earlier for a few days prior to eastward travel and an hour later for a few days prior to westward travel so your SCN will be more in line with the time at your destination.

Shift Work Sleep Disorder

About 20% of the population performs shift work, meaning they work hours outside of the normal 9–5 schedule. However, the prevalence of this reversed schedule—and its side effects—is not well recognized.

One of the most challenging side effects of shift work is shift work sleep disorder (SWSD), in which you have difficulty getting enough sleep because your schedule doesn't align with the natural day and night rhythm. You are, in a sense, fighting against nature by working at night and sleeping during the day.

The incidence of SWSD is "about 32% of night workers, 10% of daily workers and 8–26% of workers in rotating shifts."[55] It is higher in a hospital setting among nurses, medical interns, and doctors since hospitals are open 24/7. In addition, there is a shortage of healthcare workers to cover the shifts, stretching shift workers even further. SWSD is also common in factories and food-production plants that run around the clock.

The common symptoms of SWSD are daytime drowsiness (somnolence), fatigue, insomnia, and even depression. These symptoms are due to the non-synchronization of the circadian rhythm because of work schedule demands.

In the hospital setting, most shifts vary between 12 and 24 hours. Lack of sleep for such a long time, plus the absence of natural light, shifts the internal clock forward and backward, resulting in symptoms of insomnia and sleepiness.

The treatment for shift work disorder is to avoid bright light at the end of the shift, have a fixed sleep time, and if indicated, to use FDA-approved stimulant medications like modafinil and armodafinil to combat sleepiness. That being said, this is a difficult disorder to treat as the shifts vary regularly, thus placing the circadian clock under constant turmoil.

Time-Change Sleep Problems

In most states in the US, there is a change in time twice a year—once in the spring, and once in the fall. The idea behind daylight saving time (DST) is to make better use of the available daylight during the longer days of the year by shifting an hour of daylight from the morning to the evening.

While DST may be good for businesses, there are consequences to such changes due to the misalignment of your internal circadian clock. With less sunlight in the mornings during DST, there is a higher risk of accidents and workplace injuries. DST can also lead to less time spent in sleep, especially in children, with a loss of 30 minutes during weekdays, resulting in excessive daytime drowsiness and slower response times. There is also an increased incidence of heart attacks and heart rhythm irregularities associated with the first week of transition during DST.[56, 57]

For decades, there has been an ongoing debate about doing away with the time changes. While there was talk of this becoming a permanent change in the US starting November 2023, the bill had yet to be passed at the time of print.

The following tips can help with time-change issues during the transitions until the US Congress makes the final decision.

- Make sure you set your clock accordingly prior to going to sleep the night of time change.
- Prepare to go to sleep 15 minutes earlier each day for four days in a row prior to the time change in the spring, and wake up 15 minutes later each day for four days in a row prior to the time change in the fall.
- Have a fixed sleep schedule.
- Get exposure to sunlight in the mornings.
- Try to keep a good exercise regimen.
- Take a short nap during the transition period, if needed.

Fortunately, some of these sleep disorders are rare. However, I've known corporate executives who gave dismal presentations because they could not adjust to local time thanks to jet lag.

And I have seen several patients whose insomnia started after time change, and they never got back on track. Others have sleep maintenance insomnia due to awakenings due to RBD.

Still, being aware of the causes of sleeplessness allows you to address these issues, like the deleterious consequences of SRED. Likewise, being aware of the presence of RBD alerts you to the potential risk of neurological disorders like Parkinson's.

Knowledge of these disorders can help you with overall sleep quality and good health.

Chapter 4

Sleep and the Body

Pearl was a white-haired woman with deep dimples who described herself as "77 years young." When I first met her, it was obvious she was suffering from dementia. She was overweight ("pleasantly plump," according to her), had high blood pressure, diabetes, and had recently been diagnosed with Alzheimer's dementia. Her son, Reginald, a nurse practitioner, was aware that sleep apnea was one of the treatable causes of dementia, so he brought her to my office. He reported Pearl had been snoring loudly for the past several years.

Pearl was quite cheerful when we spoke, but it was obvious she had difficulty remembering recent events. She was able to vividly recount her major life events, including her marriage and college days, but she had only a faint memory of what she had for dinner last night. She had also fallen a few times in the month before coming to see me, and she attributed the falls to being tired and not having enough energy to focus.

I had her do an in-home sleep study, which showed severe sleep apnea associated with low oxygen. She also had advanced sleep phase syndrome (ASPS), a condition where bedtime is much earlier in the night than for most people. (This is more common in folks over 70.) Pearl also completed a Sleep Journal, which showed she was going to sleep at 7 p.m. and waking up at 3 a.m.

I started Pearl on CPAP therapy for her sleep apnea, and she did remarkably well. Her blood sugar and blood pressure improved. She was sleeping better and thinking more clearly. After I spoke with her about improving her sleep habits, she also started going to bed at the more appropriate time of 9:30 p.m. and waking up at 5:15 a.m.

Unfortunately, her cognitive symptoms did not improve. Her short-term memory never fully returned, and she still falls occasionally. However, I was reassured to learn that the CPAP seemed to have halted any further cognitive decline.

Reginald said he wished he had been aware of her sleep apnea earlier so that he could have prevented some of the damage, but he was glad we were able to manage her condition and keep her from deteriorating further.

Sleep and Cognition

If you've ever slept poorly, you know that your brain is a little hazy the next day. You may not be able to concentrate, forget what you were saying mid-sentence, or even make mistakes on simple tasks you normally accomplish with ease and excellence.

New moms who are up all night with newborns frequently cite "mom brain," a cognitively fuzzy state where they're forgetful and irritable due to lack of sleep. Students who are up all night for exams may report similar symptoms. Executives will also report feeling foggy during a big reorganization or important program at work.

Thankfully, most of these issues resolve once the individual can get a good night's sleep. However, for folks with chronic sleep issues like sleep apnea or insomnia, these cognitive impairments may become permanent.

That's because good sleep is crucial for healthy brain functioning.

A Lack of Sleep Is Like Being Drunk

We all know that we don't perform as well at work or school if we don't get a good night's sleep, but did you know that sleeplessness can be just as detrimental to cognition as being drunk?

A study published in *Nature* asked one group of participants to stay up all night. The other group was given varying quantities of alcohol to consume. Then, the researchers asked participants to perform a series of hand-eye coordination tests on a computer.

Not surprisingly, people scored worse on these tests the longer they had been awake. What *was* surprising was just how closely fatigue mimicked drunkenness.

The researchers described their results here:

> Equating the two rates at which performance declined (percentage decline per hour of wakefulness and percentage decline with change in blood alcohol concentration), it was evident that the performance decrement for each hour of wakefulness between 10 and 26 hours was equivalent to the performance decrement observed with a 0.004% rise in blood alcohol concentration.[58]

Another older but still relevant study found that "after 17 hours of consecutive wakefulness, participants scored roughly the same as participants with a blood alcohol concentration of 0.05%, the level considered drunk for most societies and situations."[59]

Yet another study concluded that symptoms of short-term sleep disruptions included everything from poor mood, emotional distress, increased stress, and reduced quality of life. In adults, the most noticeable issues due to sleep deprivation were diminished attention or vigilance, executive function, emotional reactivity, memory formation, decision-making, risk-taking behavior, and judgment.[60]

In adolescents, short-term sleep deprivation looked different but was still significant. For this age group, insufficient sleep was linked to declining school performance, substance abuse, and mental health problems.

Adolescents who didn't get enough sleep were much more likely to be worried, anxious, and depressed. They were also more likely to have failed or spent more years in school.[61]

For younger children, short-term sleep disruption was also detrimental. Children and teens who didn't get enough sleep had more behavioral and emotional problems than their peers who slept well.

How Sleep Protects Cognitive Function

We've established that sleep gives our brain a chance to recharge, but that's not all it does. It also allows the glymphatic system the time it needs to remove toxins so that they don't build up in the brain. One study compares this function to clearing the cobwebs, or cellular trash—every cell of our body produces waste that needs to be cleared to preserve cell function—and refreshing the brain for the next day.[62]

In other words, clarity of mind comes with sleep.

But along with clearing waste, sleep also helps us store and organize our memories. During sleep, new memories are codified and then stored in their appropriate spot, which helps us make connections, synthesize information, and learn to better predict outcomes.[63] Without sleep, we have trouble retaining new information and placing it in the context of what we already know.

Effects of Long-Term Sleep Deprivation

The link between long-term sleep disturbances and cognitive decline is well established. People with cognitive impairment or dementia are much more likely than their peers to sleep poorly.

However, researchers are beginning to realize that lack of sleep on a long-term basis can put people at risk for cognitive problems. In other words, poor sleep is not just a symptom of cognitive decline; sleeplessness and cognitive impairment have a bidirectional relationship—one makes the other worse.

Lack of sleep or irregular sleep architecture (such as if the REM to non-REM ratios is "off") can cause mild cognitive decline. Scientists believe this is because sleep helps consolidate memories, and this process can't occur if people aren't getting enough sleep—or the right kind of sleep.

Between 60–70% of people with dementia suffer from sleep disturbances, which can include short sleep duration, overly long sleep duration, and interrupted sleep. For those with Alzheimer's, the most common sleep complaints are nighttime wakefulness, frequent daytime napping, and increased confusion and restlessness in the evenings (called sundowning).[64]

Research suggests that folks who suffer from insomnia are between *two to three times more likely* to develop Alzheimer's disease. That said, researchers aren't sure if insomnia is a risk factor or a very early marker of the disease itself. Parkinson's disease is also associated with disrupted sleep, with as many as 80% of people reporting some type of sleep problem.[65]

Although the link between cognitive disorders and sleep is clear, this connection has often been overlooked. Now, doctors who are diagnosing a cognitive issue are aware to adequately examine the person's sleep pattern and consider how it may play into the progression and treatment of their disease.

In 2014, the Italian Neurological Association approved recommendations for looking more closely at sleep issues when diagnosing cognitive impairments. They recommend that sleep disorders should be "investigated using an in-depth sleep history, physical examination, questionnaires, and scales" when evaluating a person with symptoms of cognitive decline.[66] Further, they suggest that people who do have sleep irregularities be referred to a sleep specialist.

Since the causal relationship between poor sleep and cognitive decline isn't fully understood, it's important to carefully address both issues, rather than assuming one is a symptom of the other.

General Insomnia and Cognition

General insomnia that isn't caused by medical disorders or mental disorders can, unfortunately, contribute to cognitive decline. As we know, insomnia is not linked to one physiological root cause. Instead, it is usually dependent on our sleep habits, lifestyle habits, and mental health. Insomnia is usually subjective, i.e., it is self-diagnosed, but it can also be observed in a sleep study as evidenced by delay in going to sleep. Around 6–13% of the population suffers from chronic insomnia.[67]

Approximately 30% of adults worldwide report one or more symptoms of insomnia, either difficulty initiating or maintaining sleep, waking up too early, or having poor quality sleep (sleep that is not restorative).[68]

In one cognitive test, people with insomnia showed similar reaction times to their non-insomniac peers. However, they were more likely to make mistakes. Overall, researchers found that people with insomnia had mild deficits in cognitive functioning. People who complained of severe insomnia were more likely to have clinically significant cognitive declines.[69]

A 2021 study showed that specific types of insomnia are related to different forms of cognitive impairment. People with short sleep duration insomnia, i.e., who fell asleep easily enough but woke up before they'd gotten adequate rest, had more inconsistency in their cognitive function. Those with normal sleep duration insomnia, who slept a normal amount of time but had trouble going to sleep, had worse working memory and reaction times than their peers with short sleep duration insomnia or healthy sleepers.[70]

Older adults who were diagnosed with mild cognitive decline were also more likely to have insomnia-related habits that could be troublesome to the families they lived with. These nocturnal awakenings can be extremely disruptive to family life and are one of the most common reasons caretakers opt to place their parents or grandparents in nursing or assisted living facilities.

The results are clear. Whatever the cause of poor sleep, it can be quite detrimental to our cognitive health. People with mild or occasional insomnia should work on their sleep routines and seek help from a specialist if their problems persist.

People experiencing sleep apnea are even more at risk of cognitive diminishment and should make sure they're under the care of a sleep specialist.

How Poor Sleeping Shows Up in Our Bodies

Annette was a 55-year-old artist and designer who sold her paintings in some of the most exclusive art galleries in town. She worked in a world where appearances were everything. As she aged, Annette noticed the skin around her neck and arms was wrinkly, and she was concerned about the bagginess under her eyes. She was adamant about wanting a more youthful appearance, so she visited a plastic surgeon for cosmetic work.

Dr. Robbins examined her and was concerned about an irregular spot on her forehead being skin cancer. Before he would do plastic surgery, he wanted to biopsy the spot to make sure it wasn't cancerous.

Annette was apprehensive about the procedure, asking to be "knocked out." She received an anesthetic cocktail and was found snoring loudly throughout the procedure. Overall, everything went well, but Annette's oxygen levels dropped a bit. Dr. Robbins found this to be concerning.

When Annette finally woke up (taking longer than the norm), Dr. Robbins questioned his patient about her sleeping habits, mentioning the possibility of sleep apnea.

Annette reluctantly said she had gained weight recently, and her snoring was worse. She admitted that she occasionally woke up feeling like she was choking and gasping for air. That's when Dr. Robbins had her call my office.

I was able to run some tests and do an in-home sleep study and found that Annette had severe sleep apnea. I put her on a CPAP machine, and during her follow-up appointment a few months later, Annette reported that she was doing significantly better. She even noticed that the bagginess under her eyes was resolving.

Annette's skin biopsy results were negative for cancer, but she was fortunate to have survived the minor procedure to discover that she had untreated sleep apnea; patients like her are vulnerable for respiratory failure from anesthetics, hence the surgical team should be made aware of their sleep apnea so they can take necessary precautions.

☽

Sleep is such an essential process that when we go without it, the effects are obvious. You can spot someone who's struggling with sleep deprivation by just looking at them. They may be irritable, forgetful, and have dark circles under their eyes. They may be pounding energy drinks or snacking on carbs for a quick energy boost. If they're dealing with prolonged sleep issues, they may even be overweight or struggling with diabetes or hypertension.

As we know, sleep is an intricate process. But why is sleep so critical? What's the relationship, for instance, between circles or bags under the eyes and not getting a full eight hours of rest? And how does sleep deprivation affect our appetite and make us crave certain foods that lead to weight gain?

There's a direct relationship between sleep and how our body functions.

A recent study done in Japan is showing that it is not just the brain but the whole body that contributes to sleep. As you know, if you stay up for a long time, you become incredibly sleepy. The study found that the longer subjects were awake and the more active they were, the more sleep-promoting chemicals accumulated in the body tissues, resulting in falling sleep.[71] While the study was done on mice, it could be a possible mechanism in humans too.

We have always known that farmers, hard laborers, and folks who exercise a lot had the soundest sleep, and this could be the plausible mechanism. I am excited about studies such as this to be expanded to humans.

The Brain: Memory, Dreaming, and Learning

Even though the millions of neurons in the brain slow down during sleep, they're still performing important work. Learning and memory processing are some of the most important benefits of good sleep.

Let's say that you're a college student, and you listen to a lecture during the day. While you may pay close attention, you still need a good night of sleep to consolidate what you've learned. It's as if the facts you heard at the lecture are in a pile on the floor, waiting to be appropriately organized into the right filing cabinets. When you sleep, your brain decides where each memory should be stored and places it in the correct spot so that you can access it the next time you are awake. If you don't get a good night's sleep after the lecture, the information you learned could be forgotten entirely.

When I see children who struggle with learning, I check their sleep habits first. Although most memory consolidation happens during REM cycles, non-REM sleep is also needed for brain functioning. During non-REM sleep, the brain decides which memories to keep and which to toss. Once the brain has selected the keeper memories, it will further consolidate them during sleep.

Often people who are sleep-deprived will say they are in a brain fog and cannot get their thoughts together. This is because the normal processes haven't had the chance to happen, for memory storing, attention, and concentration. When a person has a long-term sleep disorder like sleep apnea that goes untreated, serious memory impairment—even dementia—can result.

Maintaining healthy sleep habits also affects performance, and several studies have shown the harmful effects of sleep deprivation on attention, concentration, and executive functioning.

There are several neurological conditions that can be better treated by improving sleep quality and treating associated sleep disorders. These include stroke, uncontrolled epilepsy or seizure disorder, Parkinson's, muscular weakness, autism, and uncontrollable headaches.

Sleep and Immune Function

If you've ever endured a period of poor sleep, you've probably noticed that you tend to get sick much more often. That's because sleep is crucial for boosting the immune system. Without sleep, the T-cells—part of our immune system that helps protect us from infection—cannot perform their duty of defending the body from germs. This leaves your body much more vulnerable to common viruses and bacterial infections. For example, you may notice you're more likely to come down coughing and sniffling after a long trip where you didn't get much sleep.

There are several studies that indicate markers of inflammation in the body, like interleukins, are elevated in long-term sufferers of insomnia and sleep apnea.[72] (Interleukins are proteins that the white blood cells produce. Several interleukins are good; they fight infections and protect our bodies, while others can be hurtful.)

Sleep and Growth

During the first few hours of sleep, especially the first cycle each night of slow-wave sleep, the pituitary gland secretes more HGH (human growth hormone, as you may recall) than any other time. HGH promotes growth in every tissue, especially the bones in children and adolescents.

That's why it's crucial for infants and young children to get adequate sleep. Lack of sleep may stunt their development.

Once the growth plates are fused, we no longer grow. Still, HGH is involved in regulation of blood sugar by causing the liver to produce insulin. So, even as adults, we need HGH to maintain healthy blood sugar levels, support our metabolism, and maintain our body's structure.

Sleep and the Lungs

Our lungs function by filtering our blood and providing oxygen to the body. Breathing is controlled by the brain's respiratory center in the medulla.

We breathe about 14–16 times per minute when awake, and while sleeping, it slows to about 12–14 times. In REM sleep, breathing can become irregular. This makes people with lung problems like COPD (emphysema) more vulnerable during this sleep stage.

Poor sleep compounds the risk for asthma in adults as noted in the *British Medical Journal.* The researchers saw a 47–55% higher incidence of asthma in poor sleepers when they were followed for eight years. They attributed it to poor-sleep-induced chronic inflammation contributing to the exacerbation of asthma.[73]

The study concluded that having better sleeping habits could prevent future asthma attacks in patients who are genetically prone to develop asthma.

Folks with sleep apnea are more vulnerable to sedatives and anesthetics as these medications can cause suppression of the respiratory center, which in turn can cause the tissues around the throat to relax, resulting in a narrowing of the throat, and leading to a potential dramatic drop in oxygen levels. (Like what happened with Annette.)

For this reason, when planning any procedure that requires sedation or anesthesia, anyone with sleep apnea should make sure to inform their surgical team.

Sleep and the Skin

By now, you know that melatonin is a naturally occurring hormone that induces sleep. But did you know that melatonin is also essential for your skin? Melatonin protects the skin from environmental and endogenous (or internal) stressors.

If your body isn't releasing melatonin at night—whether because of artificial light or the use of a chemical sleep aid—your skin won't get the help it needs. That can lead the skin to lose elasticity, leading to wrinkles, dark circles, and bags under your eyes.

It is easy to recognize a person who has poor sleep by noticing their "raccoon eyes." Their skin has lost its elasticity and structural integrity because it hasn't been getting the melatonin it needs to guard against stressors.

In fact, a study published in the *Journal of Clinical Dermatology* sought to answer the question: "Does poor sleep quality affect skin aging?" The researchers looked at people with poor quality sleep who were subjected to solar ultraviolet light. The recovery of the redness of the skin was assessed and compared to healthy sleepers. It was clear that good sleepers had a 30% better recovery rate than poor sleepers in 72 hours.[74] The study also showed poor sleepers had signs of skin aging, diminished skin protection function, and lower satisfaction with their appearances.

Sleep, Blood Pressure, and the Cardiovascular System

If you struggle with high blood pressure, you're not alone. About 75 million Americans—or one in three adults—have hypertension, and high blood pressure is one of the leading risks for heart disease and stroke.

During normal sleep, your blood pressure should decrease. It's natural for your blood pressure to be higher during the day, when you're dealing with stressors, but it's supposed to auto-regulate and decrease at night when you're asleep and relaxed. Except, this reset does not happen if you're not resting well.

If you suffer from poor sleep or a sleep disorder, your blood pressure stays higher at night. In the case of sleep apnea, the interruption of oxygen causes a constant release of hormones such as norepinephrine as a fight-or-flight response. This, in turn, causes the heart to pump faster and harder and the blood vessels to narrow, resulting in higher blood pressure at night.

During REM sleep, pulse and blood pressure can be variable, sometimes triggering arrhythmias, especially in people with cardiovascular conditions.

Sleep apnea needs to be ruled out in most people diagnosed with high blood pressure or cardiac conditions, like an irregular heart rate (atrial fibrillation) or a history of heart attacks.

Untreated sleep apnea is one of the most common causes of uncontrolled hypertension. But by treating their sleep apnea, patients may find that they can also be weaned off their blood pressure medications. Control of blood pressure also reduces their chances of a stroke or heart attack.

Meanwhile, there is a strong association between severe untreated sleep apnea and persistently elevated blood pressure despite aggressive treatment with blood pressure medications. For this reason, I cannot emphasize enough how important it is to test patients who have high blood pressure to see if they might also have sleep apnea that needs to be treated. [75]

Personally, I've had many patients come off multiple blood pressure medications by addressing their sleep problems.

Untreated sleep apnea has also been linked to other cardiovascular disorders that can lead to blood vessel damage and the buildup of fats and cholesterol—a condition called atherosclerosis.[76] This plaque buildup can cause arteries to narrow, which obstructs blood flow and can result in a heart attack.

Sleep and the Musculoskeletal System

How our bodies work when we sleep is truly remarkable. Our entire musculoskeletal system is relaxed during sleep, especially in REM sleep when most of the muscles are paralyzed (called atonia) except for the diaphragm and eye muscles. This full-body relaxation gives the muscles time to repair and rebuild from the previous day and prepare for the day ahead. It also promotes healing.

Not surprisingly, there is a correlation between sleep deprivation and chronic pain conditions like fibromyalgia, most likely because the muscles don't have the opportunity to recover and relax fully during sleep.

Sleep and the Endocrine System

Sleep and the body's internal clock—your circadian rhythm—play an important role in regulating the production of numerous hormones. Quality sleep is very important in optimal secretion of melatonin, HGH, leptin, and ghrelin, among others. Melatonin promotes sleep and skin integrity, and human growth hormones help with growth, metabolism, and blood sugar control.

Leptin and ghrelin play an important role in regulating appetite, which is why sleep deprivation can lead to weight gain and even diabetes.

Our hormone levels fluctuate during different sleep stages, and the quality of sleep may also affect your daytime hormone production.[77] If you don't get enough sleep at night, your daytime hormone levels may also suffer. Lack of sleep can also release stress hormones that can result in weight gain, predisposing you to diabetes.

Sleep and Diabetes

Sadly, diabetes is on the rise with devastating impact.

Diabetes is a disorder in which your pancreas either produces inadequate insulin or your body does not respond appropriately to insulin hormone, that is, you are insulin resistant.

Uncontrolled blood sugar over time damages small blood vessels throughout the body. This damage ultimately affects multiple organs like the eyes, kidneys, stomach, nervous system, and skin. This organ failure can even lead to blindness and amputation.

Diabetes is classified as type 1 and type 2.

Type 1 is due to the lack of insulin produced by the pancreas from a young age. It is also called juvenile or insulin-dependent diabetes and most often shows up at a young age. The exact cause is unknown, but it is believed to be caused by an autoimmune disorder or viral infection that destroys the insulin-making cells in the pancreas.

Type 2 is more common in adults when the body can no longer use insulin properly. The pancreas is making adequate insulin, but the tissues are resistant and not able to process it, thus resulting in elevated blood sugars.

So, what's the relationship between sleep and diabetes? As we saw earlier, poor sleep can increase the flow of stress hormones and can affect the flow of hormones that regulate appetite, thus resulting in weight gain and poorly controlled diabetes.

And when sleep-deprived and wanting a quick burst of energy, people also tend to make poorer food choices—like reaching for simple carbs (processed foods) and sugary treats (like cakes and cookies) instead of lean proteins.

On the other hand, adequate sleep and good sleep strategies help to curb bad eating habits and help your body regulate sugars.

So please hear this: If you have poorly controlled diabetes, please get a sleep evaluation to rule out sleep disorders, specifically sleep apnea. Not only will this help improve your sleep quality, but it could also save your life!

Good sleep motivates you, boosts your energy levels, and makes it easier to have a consistent regimen. When you're active, sleeping and eating right, it's much easier to maintain your blood sugar.

Sleep and the Thyroid

Interestingly, the thyroid is one of the few hormones *not* produced in sleep.

The functioning of the thyroid gland is a classic example of the delicate interaction between the circadian rhythm and sleep. The thyroid gland is under the influence of thyroid stimulating hormone (TSH), which is secreted by the master endocrine controller, the pituitary gland.

TSH under circadian influence is maximally stimulated in the evening and prior to sleep onset. It decreases during sleep and is completely turned off in deep sleep, giving the thyroid a rest. However, sleep deprivation and frequent awakening results in increased secretion of TSH at night, thus altering thyroid function.[78]

When you sleep poorly, it affects more than your energy levels. It contributes to cognition and memory challenges, upsets endocrine hormone secretion and immune function, and impacts *every* system in the body. That is why it's *so* important to foster healthy sleep habits. Among other benefits, it can help prevent conditions like diabetes even before they start.

Chapter 5

Sleep and Mental Health

Jenni was a 21-year-old college student who wanted to end it all. She had recently attempted suicide by an overdose of pills, but, fortunately, her roommate found her in the nick of time.

After she was resuscitated, Jenni was admitted to the ICU and was then transferred to an in-patient psychiatric facility for further evaluation and management.

When asked about her medical history, Jenni cried uncontrollably, explaining that since she was 13 years old, she had struggled with a severe eating disorder and significant fatigue.

Once she was stable, a psychiatrist evaluated Jenni and prescribed multiple medications. Sadly, none of it helped. After considering Jenni's issues with chronic fatigue, the psychiatrist suspected that Jenni might have a sleep disorder, so he referred Jenni to my clinic.

Jenni's mom accompanied her for the first consultation, and she shared that her daughter had been having problems since middle school because she was always sleepy. Her mom attributed Jenni's exhaustion to her busy cheerleading schedule and school workload, but I suspected something else was going on.

Jenni mentioned that under stress or emotional extremes, she felt weak in her knees and frequently dropped objects. She also had significant hallucinations, which she had attributed to a medication she had been taking to treat her depression.

Over the past decade, Jenni had lost interest in sports and other fun activities because she always felt tired. Even more concerning, Jenni stated that she sometimes had difficulty waking up in the morning because she felt she couldn't move, a condition called sleep paralysis that is frequently seen in people with narcolepsy.

I sent her to the sleep lab, and with further testing it became clear that she had the classic diagnostic criteria for narcolepsy.

I prescribed Jenni a stimulant medication, which significantly improved her symptoms. It's been a few years now, and Jenni continues to do well. She was weaned off her depression medications but still follows up with her psychiatrist periodically and is enjoying life again.

This is an extreme case of fatigue from a sleep disorder masquerading as depression—and a reminder to look into secondary causes of depression.

Sleep and Psychological Health

Often, significant daytime fatigue and hypersomnia (being sleepy all the time) can be mistaken for depression. Disrupted sleep can make you feel like you're trapped in a vicious cycle you can't escape with one problem feeding another. However, understanding the relationship between sleep deprivation and depression can help manage both conditions better.

In an ideal situation, our sleep and our mental health function hand in hand, with both processes nourishing and supporting each other. Good sleep helps us stay healthy psychologically, and staying healthy psychologically helps us get good sleep.

Unfortunately, for many of my patients this symbiotic relationship has gotten off track. When either sleep or mental health falters, it impacts the other, thus creating a spiraling effect.

My good friend, psychiatrist Dr. Sricharan Moturi, describes the correlation between sleep and mental health as bidirectional, meaning it functions in both directions.

Anxiety and depression can cause poor sleep, and poor sleep can worsen symptoms of anxiety and depression. But improving your sleep can also help your mental health, and improving your mental health can improve your sleep quality.

Many sleep disorders, such as insomnia and nightmares, have a psychological component. And severe depression has been associated with insomnia and daytime sleepiness. Similarly, severe anxiety can also create difficulty falling asleep or can even trigger nocturnal panic attacks in some people.[79]

Other psychiatric disorders like ADHD and its near twin, ADD (attention-deficit disorder), have been associated with primary sleep disorders like OSA and RLS, especially in children.

Dr. Moturi recommends getting a sleep history to determine the quality and duration of sleep for every psychiatric patient, plus a thorough physical examination to rule out disorders like sleep apnea and RLS.

When sleep issues are resolved, less psychiatric medications are generally needed, and overall psychiatric outcomes improve in both adults and children, warding off future relapses. For this reason, **I cannot stress highly enough how important good sleep habits are—for both treating mental illness and warding off a future relapse.**

While mental illness is beyond the scope of this book, I will briefly touch on some of the most common psychological disorders and how they affect sleep.

Anxiety and Sleep

Anxiety is a natural part of being human. We're meant to feel afraid or worried in dangerous situations. Stress and anxiety trigger our bodies to release cortisol that helps us react quickly to escape harm (fight-or-flight response).[80] But if you have chronic anxiety, you might feel stress or worry all the time. You may feel fearful of everyday situations like driving to work or even falling asleep.

Chronically high levels of cortisol, especially before sleep, can make it hard for your body to relax. You may have difficulty falling asleep. If you do fall asleep, you may wake up during the night with stressful or worrisome thoughts and not be able to fall asleep again.

Every one of us deals with stress most days, and most of us experience extreme stress at some point in our lives. But with anxiety, this distress becomes excessive.[81] The fears we experience are sometimes not proportional to the situation—they seem larger than life—and worry interferes with our daily tasks and routine. These negative and frustrating feelings become persistent, occurring most days and for a period of several months or even longer.

Anxiety is a catch-all term, but there are varying degrees of anxiety, from general anxiety to panic attacks and phobias. Physically, anxiety disorders can often provoke tense muscles, rapid breathing, elevated heartbeat, sweating, trembling, gastrointestinal distress, and fatigue.

Anxiety is frequently connected to a multitude of sleeping problems. Excessive worry and fear make it harder for us to turn off our racing thoughts, which prevents us from falling asleep or staying asleep through the night.

Sleep deprivation can, in turn, worsen anxiety, creating a vicious cycle between the two. Sleep disorders also cause daytime sleepiness and fatigue, and this exhaustion results in worsening anxiety symptoms.

Though sleep deprivation can certainly make anxiety worse, it's difficult to identify one root cause for all anxiety disorders. Family history, genetics, and negative life events—especially those in early life—can all play a role in setting up a person for anxiety.

Anxiety disorders are the most common type of mental illness in the US,[82] affecting the lives of an estimated 31.1% of adults, and 31.9% of teenagers between 13 and 18. [83]

The everyday impact of anxiety can vary from person to person. In one survey, around 43% of adults[84] described anxiety as causing at least a mild disruption in their life. Around 33% said it was moderate, with almost 23% saying their anxiety was severe. [85]

Anxiety is one of the leading causes of disturbed or insufficient sleep. Folks with anxiety are in a state of mental hyperarousal—an abnormal state of increased responsiveness, frequently marked by persistent worry.

Also, when people get a lot of *wrong* information about good sleep, and this adds to their anxiety before bedtime. That's why I tell all my clients that once they have seen me in consultation, they should quit reading about insomnia or sleep-related topics.

Stress remains one of the biggest enemies of sleep. It causes excessive worry and rumination, which can make it more difficult to fall asleep, while also elevating cortisol levels, causing fragmentation of the normal sleep architecture. There are a number of causes for stress, including personal, professional, academic, and financial pressures. These stressors vary with life stage but are often impossible to fully resolve, which is why it's so important to implement effective coping mechanisms.

But there are ways to help with stress—meditation, yoga, Vivid Imagination®, and exercise can all make a difference. Removing triggers like smartphones, computers, and TVs from the bedroom can also help lessen stress. If you're unable to fully get a handle on your stress after changing your lifestyle, it may be worth seeing a therapist or other mental health professional.

Hyperarousal has also been identified as a key factor behind difficulty in initiating and maintaining sleep. This simply means that *people with anxiety disorders are at a higher risk for developing insomnia* and are inclined to have an increased number of sleep disruptions, so they are more likely to have sleeping problems when they are faced with stressful situations.

It's not unusual for sleep to be fragmented, and normal awakenings due to noise or needing to use the restroom are typical, but sleep fragmentation can be exaggerated in people with anxiety. While a person without anxiety can easily fall back asleep after waking up, for example to use the restroom, a person with anxiety may stay awake for hours after, watching the clock and worrying that they won't be able to fall back asleep.

When anxiety persists, it will often prevent someone from falling asleep or staying asleep for any restful period of time, so when morning comes, they are exhausted and frustrated from the lack of restorative sleep.

Anxiety also changes sleep cycles. Anxiety and worry may especially affect REM or dream sleep. Anxiety can provoke more disturbing dreams and create a higher likelihood of sleep fragmentation.

Anxiety symptoms could also prevent people from entering deep sleep; instead, they get poor and non-restorative sleep, which in turn worsens the symptoms of anxiety. Each condition makes the other one worse.

The good news is that *anxiety is treatable.* If you're experiencing disruptive levels of fear, worry, and stress, consult your physician to get the help you need.

Sleep Anxiety

Fear about falling asleep (also called sleep anxiety) can itself complicate matters, creating anxiety that reinforces a person's sense of angst and preoccupation around bedtime. In folks suffering from a long-term inability to go to sleep or stay asleep, the thought of going to bed can be anxiety provoking in and of itself. This turns their mind into high gear, causing *anxiety about getting to sleep and staying asleep*, which is counterproductive.

Waking up day after day exhausted after not sleeping for weeks on end can lead to fear of even going to bed at night. The sense of dread that you're not going to be able to sleep and will be miserable the next day is brutal. Obviously, worrying about not sleeping can create a negative loop that is counterproductive to healthy sleep.

Constant rumination (when you feel stuck in a cycle of negative thoughts) further affects the ability to sleep. Most people who are poor sleepers also have anxiety. As with sleep and general mental health, sleep and anxiety share a bidirectional relationship. By getting your sleep in order, the anxiety symptoms can improve.

Sleep and Depression

It's not surprising that, like anxiety, depression is often linked to poor sleep.

Again, being human, we all experience feelings of sadness, disappointment, loss, and grief. But depression is characterized by *excessive* feelings of loss or sadness. It can also manifest as extreme fatigue or a lack of interest in normal activities that the person once enjoyed.

According to the United Nations, the estimated number of people living with depression is over 300 million.[86] Of those, most also suffer from insomnia. The more severe the depression, the more severe the insomnia.

ABC News recently reported that up to seven out of 10 people with poor sleep also suffer from depression.[87] Depression and insomnia can aggravate each other, sometimes creating a devastating domino effect.

Depression and insomnia are, as we discussed earlier, bidirectional, meaning they make each other worse. Depression makes it harder to sleep, and people already suffering from insomnia carry at least twice the risk of developing depression than those who sleep normally.

In an article on the link between sleep and depression, journalist Lauren Krouse points out, "Since insomnia has been identified as a risk factor for depression, researchers believe diagnosing and treating sleep issues early on could possibly help lower the risk of developing depression."[88]

This is another area where you may think being depressed is somehow your fault because you can't pull yourself up by the bootstraps to feel better. But, in fact, one of the reasons why chronic lack of sleep can lead to depression is due to the reduced secretion of a crucial neurotransmitter in the brain called serotonin.

Serotonin helps regulate your attention, behavior, digestion, blood flow, and mood, among other things. Without an adequate supply of serotonin, you might feel sad, tired, or depressed. **If you don't get enough sleep, your body's production of serotonin will decrease, causing a cascade of problems. One of the most serious of these problems is depression.**

When a person is experiencing depression and insomnia, I recommend they address the problem from both ends and *treat depression and insomnia at the same time.*

Consultation with a psychiatrist or psychologist, lifestyle modification, cognitive behavioral therapy (CBT), and medication management can all help prevent and mitigate depression. If medication is needed, genetic testing can help your doctor choose the right antidepressant for you.

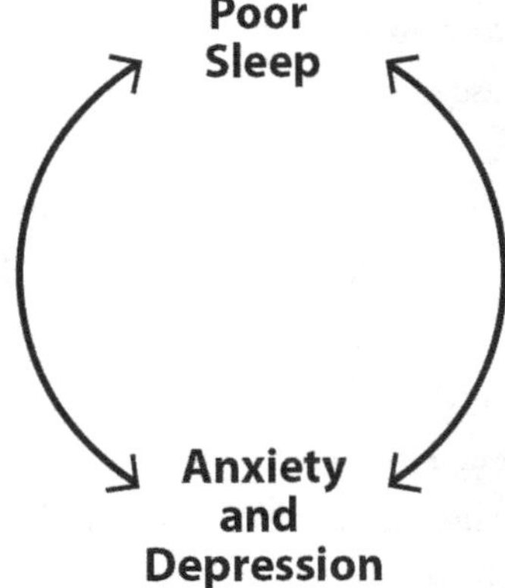

FIGURE 4. The Connection between Sleep, Anxiety, and Depression

Post-Traumatic Stress Disorder

Many people experience trauma at some point in their lives. After experiencing or witnessing a traumatic event, however, some develop PTSD. It can affect individuals from all walks of life, including military personnel, survivors of natural disasters, victims of violence, or those who have undergone severe emotional or physical trauma.

People with PTSD often experience distressing symptoms such as flashbacks, nightmares, intense anxiety, and a persistent sense of fear or danger. They may also exhibit avoidance behaviors, detachment from loved ones, and emotional numbing.

Most folks with PTSD also have restless sleep, flashbacks, vivid dreams, and nightmares. Sleep studies show diminished total sleep time, reduced deep sleep, increased awakenings, excessive movement, and REM sleep fragmentation.

For anyone with PTSD, particularly if they have symptoms of snoring or abnormal movements in their sleep, a sleep study should be part of their treatment to determine whether there are any underlying sleep disorders like sleep apnea, PLMD, or RBD.

As disruptive as PTSD is to sleep, several treatments have shown great effectiveness in treating this disorder. Medications like prazosin have been used widely—and with great success—to help with nightmare symptoms associated with PTSD.

I always recommend that anyone struggling with PTSD consult with a psychologist or psychiatrist who specializes in this area. These professionals can offer behavioral therapies, prescribe medications, or present other treatment options essential to helping people cope with severe trauma.

Alcohol and Insomnia

Alcohol is often used to help us relax. Because alcohol has sedative properties, there are many folks who use alcohol to fall asleep, but it doesn't promote healthy sleep as many people believe.

Initially, alcohol affects the portion of the brain called the prefrontal cortex and releases the restraints, which is why folks feel uninhibited and relaxed when drinking. As the intake increases, you move from tipsy to inebriated. Consume too much alcohol and you can even pass out.

But alcohol-induced sleep is not natural sleep as it does not trigger the release of sleep-promoting chemicals. Instead, it has an anesthetic effect on the brain by *mimicking* sleep. It simply drowns the brain. That's why alcohol-induced sleep is neither deep nor restful. This is *not* the ideal way to initiate sleep.

To make matters worse, alcohol is metabolized by the liver and releases a chemical called acetaldehyde that results in awakening, confusion, even combativeness.

Plus, alcohol is a diuretic, making you use the restroom more frequently, and this can result in dehydration. So, it's no wonder folks wake up feeling hungover and not rested after a night of drinking.

Not only that, but you can also quickly develop a dependency on alcohol to fall asleep. That means you'll need more and more drinks to create the same effect as you build up a tolerance, thus creating an addiction.

Sleep Disturbances and Relationships

Poor sleep has a tremendous influence on our relationships in general. We spend a third of our lives in the bedroom, which should be a place of tranquility and comfort. And when one isn't sleeping due to a partner snoring or tossing and turning, the one most frustrated by the situation might leave the bedroom, opting for the couch or spare bedroom just to get away from the disturbance, thus resulting in a sleep divorce.

It's no surprise that sleep deprivation has an impact on intimacy—the lack of sleep can be exhausting and often results in not having enough energy for sex. When you are rested you are more patient and have more energy, and the chemistry between couples is much better. This may be reason enough for some couples to seek treatment.

In a similar way, simple interactions with those we love and work with can be severely taxed when we are too tired. Being snippy is often a sign of being exhausted and not having energy—often, as direct result of poor sleep.

Sleep and Cell Phones

Since the first iPhone came on the market in 2007, cell phones have changed how we live life. For the most part, for the better. But cell phones can also interfere with sleep, and out-of-control cell phone use can have devastating consequences for how we live our lives.

Unfortunately, cell phone addiction can profoundly disrupt our sleep patterns and sleep quality. The constant use of smartphones, especially right before bedtime, exposes us to the stimulating effects of blue light emitted by screens. This blue light suppresses the production of melatonin, the hormone responsible for regulating sleep–wake cycles, making it more difficult to fall asleep. The light from the cell phone also relays signals to the brain that it's still daytime and there is no need to sleep.

Moreover, the habitual checking of messages, social media updates, or playing games on our phones can lead to increased anxiety and stress, further hindering our ability to unwind and relax before sleep.

Additionally, notifications throughout the night can disrupt the deep and restorative stages of sleep, causing frequent awakenings and reducing the overall quality of rest we get. In the long run, this addiction can result in chronic sleep deprivation, which has detrimental effects on our physical and mental health, including impaired cognitive function and increased risk of various health conditions.

It's essential to recognize the effect cell phone addiction has on our sleep and take steps to establish healthier bedtime routines for the sake of our (and our children's) well-being.

Breaking cell phone addiction can be challenging, but with persistence and the right strategies, it is possible to regain control over phone usage.

Here are some effective ways to break cell phone addiction:

Recognize the problem: Acknowledge that you have an addiction to your cell phone and that it is negatively impacting your life. Picking up the phone first thing in the morning is one sign that you are addicted. Recognizing the problem is the first step toward finding a solution.

Set clear goals: Define specific goals for reducing phone usage. This could include limiting screen time, designating certain phone-free periods, or establishing boundaries for phone use in social situations.

Create a schedule: Develop a daily or weekly schedule that allocates specific times for phone use and times for other activities. Stick to the schedule as much as possible, and gradually decrease the time allocated for phone use over time.

Remove tempting apps: Identify the apps that contribute most to your phone addiction, such as social media or games, and consider deleting or disabling them. You can also use app blockers or limiters to restrict access to certain apps during specific periods.

Establish phone-free zones: Designate certain areas or times where phones are completely off-limits. For example, establish phone-free mealtimes to enhance social interactions, and you can ban phones from the bedroom to promote better sleep.

Find alternative activities: Engage in activities that are fulfilling and enjoyable to replace excessive phone use. This could include hobbies, exercise, reading, spending time with loved ones, or pursuing personal goals.

Practice mindfulness: Cultivate mindfulness to become more aware of your phone usage habits and the impact they have on your well-being. Mindfulness exercises such as meditation or deep breathing can help reduce the impulse to constantly check your phone.

Use phone-tracking tools: There are various apps available that can track your phone usage and provide insights into your habits. Monitoring your usage can help you become more aware of the amount of time spent on your phone and motivate you to make changes.

Seek support: Share your goal of breaking phone addiction with supportive friends, family, or a support group. They can provide encouragement, accountability, and help you stay on track.

Practice self-discipline: Develop self-discipline by resisting the urge to check your phone constantly. Start by setting small, achievable goals, and gradually increase the duration of time you spend away from your phone.

Prioritize self-care: Take care of your physical and mental well-being. Get sufficient sleep, exercise regularly, eat a balanced diet, and engage in activities that reduce stress. When you feel good, you are less likely to rely on your phone for comfort or distraction.

Remember that breaking an addiction takes time and effort, and setbacks are normal. Be patient with yourself and celebrate small victories along the way. With perseverance and commitment, you can regain control over your phone usage and live a more balanced and fulfilling life—and wake refreshed after a deep and restorative sleep.

The Role of Mental Health Professionals

While I often refer to the fact that I get many referrals from mental health professionals, the reverse is also true—I see people who get their sleep issues under control, but they don't know how to fix the psychological damage that's been done so I refer them to mental health professionals.

There's much to be said for seeking out mental health professionals at all different levels, depending on what your concerns are. For example, it may be appropriate to look into seeing a psychiatrist for diagnosing and treating mental disorders.

A marriage and family therapist could also help with communication or other problems that have come up over the years. A licensed counselor can be a good person to discuss stress issues, work issues, and life issues to help get perspective on the many challenges we all face in life.

The body, mind, and sleep connection is very evident. All three must function cohesively for us to be at our best. They are mutually inclusive.

Mental health and physical health work hand in hand for us to get a good night's sleep.

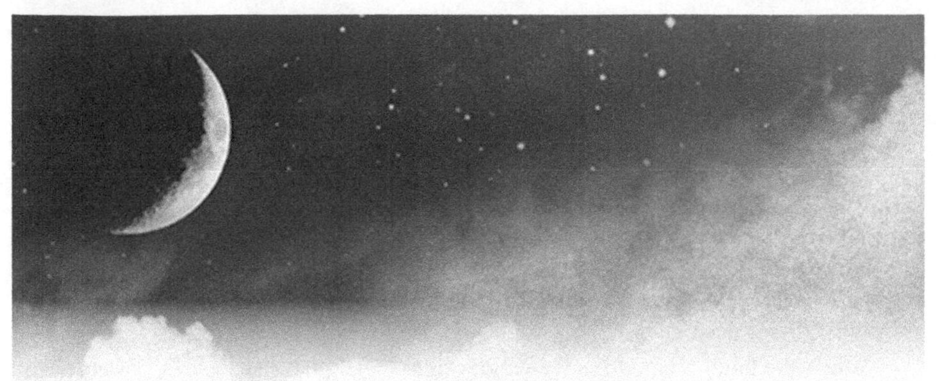

Chapter 6

Sleep, Weight Gain, and Weight Loss

Sue, approaching age 70, met with me and told me she had struggled with her weight and sleep issues all her life.

When she was in junior high school, her mom took her to her first "diet workshop" meeting to learn how to eat right and control her weight. In fact, Sue remembers her mom saying, "You're *always* going to have to watch eating those mashed potatoes, honey. . ."

She wasn't technically obese, but she always knew that she was a little heavier than her peers.

When Sue got to college, she stayed up late to study and cram for exams, often slept in in the mornings, and quickly put on the "freshman 15."

After she married and got pregnant, Sue gained 25 pounds more than her doctor's suggested goal weight for her first pregnancy, and after the baby's birth, she gained "a bit more" due to being up all night with her newborn. She eventually got her weight back down, and then repeated the process with her second baby.

As life went on, between babies, kids, teens, work, hormones, stress, worries, and the ups and downs of life, Sue would always lose weight, gain the weight back, go on some new diet, lose weight, only to gain it back again in a "lather, rinse, repeat" cycle.

Deep down, Sue believed that her chronic weight struggles were because of a lack of self-control and falling off the rails when it came to food. Her self-esteem would plummet and, once again, and she'd find herself trapped in a vicious loop where she couldn't seem to break the pattern.

All the while, Sue was also frustrated with not sleeping well and always feeling tired.

When she finally came to see me about her challenging sleep issues, I wasn't at all surprised when she also shared about her lifelong struggle with her weight.

When I asked her when she first remembered having sleep issues, Sue recalled being just 11 or 12 years old and getting out of bed to go and watch the late-night shows on TV with her dad because she couldn't sleep. And in college, she would stay up late studying, but then she just couldn't pull herself out of bed for an 8 a.m. class.

Now, decades later, I was successfully able to treat her sleep issues and she was surprised to find that when she was able to sleep better, she was also able to get her weight down—and keep it down.

Is Poor Sleeping Making Us Fat?

There is an epidemic of obesity in America and around the world. According to data from the CDC looking at 2017 to March 2020, 41.9% of Americans were obese, which was up from 30.6% in 1999. By 2019, the annual medical cost of obesity-related illness in the US was $173 *billion* dollars.[89]

So, what is causing this obesity epidemic? Many factors contribute to this crisis, but let's look at how sleep, in particular, plays a role in weight regulation.

Just like we saw with mental health, sleep and weight gain have a complicated relationship. Insomnia can lead us to eat more and gain weight, and being overweight can cause sleep disorders like OSA.

Take, for instance, eating habits. Studies demonstrate that increased food intake in the evenings can negatively impact our sleep patterns, especially our sleep quality. High-caloric food intake before bed is correlated with increased sleep latency—the time it takes to fall asleep.

One study showed that when volunteers consumed a meal only 30–60 minutes before they went to bed, their sleep was notably worse.[90] Staying up late also results in increased calorie intake because the longer we're awake, the more often we might decide to grab a late-night snack. Metabolism is slowed in sleep, so these habits of eating more food before bed result in increased weight gain.

Another study proves that food quality, not just timing, affects sleep.[91] High-fat and high-glycemic index foods—think soft drinks, sugary foods, white bread, white rice, potatoes, and potato chips—eaten before bed are also associated with increased sleep latency.

The glycemic index is a measure of how each food affects your blood sugar after it's consumed. High-protein foods like meat or beans have a low glycemic index, while simple carbohydrates like bread or candy have a high glycemic index.

Studies have demonstrated that individuals who ingested a high-glycemic index meal—even as long as four hours prior to sleep—had a harder time falling asleep.[92] On the other hand, studies show that meals with a lower glycemic index can sometimes shorten sleep latency or make it easier to fall asleep, provided these meals aren't eaten close to bedtime.[93] And a high intake of fat was associated with a lower sleep duration and more napping during the day.

For this reason, I recommend my clients to steer clear of simple carbs and fatty foods before bed. If you're going to eat a meal that has a higher glycemic index, consider eating it for lunch instead of dinner.

How much you eat also impacts your sleep. You've probably noticed that if you eat too much at dinner, it's more difficult to fall asleep. It may be tempting to go back for seconds or thirds or to clear your plate at a restaurant instead of taking home any leftovers, but a few hours later, when you're still uncomfortably full, you may regret your choice. High gastric volume, otherwise known as the sensation of being *too full*, causes discomfort, thus affecting sleep.

This can lead to a vicious cycle as sleeping poorly, in turn, can cause you to eat more. In addition to eating more food late at night because you're bored or craving a snack, according to a recent study, poor sleep increases the body's production of cortisol.[94]

Cortisol, called the stress hormone, can result in stress eating, which can result in poor food choices and craving high-calorie, high-fat foods, thus causing you to gain more weight.

Certain drugs—even some used to treat depression—can also cause an increased appetite.

The Relationship Between Sleep and Obesity in Children

Sadly, obesity is not just an adult problem. According to the CDC, 19.7% of children in the US are considered obese. That amounts to about 14.7 million American children.[95]

As with adults, there are many factors that contribute to these startling statistics, including socioeconomic status and genetic tendencies. However, in my opinion, sleep is one of the most overlooked factors in this epidemic.

Reports from a Japanese study with a sample of over eight thousand children aged 6–7 found out there was correlation between short-sleeping hours (less than eight hours) and childhood obesity. Compared with children who had 10 or more hours of sleep, children who got fewer than 10 hours of sleep had a 1.49% higher chance of developing obesity. For children who get fewer than eight hours a night, that number went up to 2.87%.[96]

Another study published in 2020 in *Pediatrics* found that "young children who routinely stayed up late (after 9 p.m.) tended to gain more body fat between 2 and 6 years old. These children had bigger increases in waist size and body mass index (BMI) compared to kids with earlier bedtimes."[97, 98]

One of the reasons for the weight gain included eating high-glycemic foods late at night, closer to bedtime. It's easy to see how these behavioral patterns developed in childhood or the teenage years can easily carry into adulthood with the same results.

How Does Poor Sleep Affect Weight?

So, now that we've established the connection between poor sleep and weight gain, let's look at *how* this relationship occurs.

We know that chronic sleep deprivation results in weight gain by increasing caloric intake and decreasing energy burn, i.e., slowing down the metabolism, but let's break this down further.

First, sleep deprivation changes the ratio of our hormones. It is well known that sleep deprivation results in an increase of the appetite-stimulating hormone called ghrelin. At the same time, sleep deprivation causes a decrease in the production of leptin, a hormone that suppresses our hunger. That means, the more sleep you miss, the hungrier you'll feel.

There is also a tendency in sleep-deprived folks to crave foods rich in fat and carbohydrates (those high-glycemic foods we mentioned earlier). In other words, since you're not getting the energy from sleeping and resting well, you look for it in high-calorie foods.

Plus, people who are sleep-deprived tend to snack more during the extra hours they are awake. This behavior is also very common in people who work the night shift, alternate between day and night shifts, or who travel a lot. They tend to have an irregular meal pattern, make bad food choices, and increase their intake of fast food and high-calorie food.

People who don't get adequate sleep are also more tired, and thus, are less inclined to make exercise a priority during the day. Instead, they spend more time watching TV or playing video games. With chronic sleep deprivation, there is also a trend toward lowering core body temperature, and this, in turn, slows the metabolism even further.

In short, adequate sleep and good sleep hygiene practices help to curb bad eating habits. Good sleep motivates you and gives you extra energy to work out. If you maintain consistent, healthy sleep strategies, you'll develop a regimen that helps keep your food intake and energy expenditure formula at an equilibrium. In other words, getting good sleep ensures you're not eating more calories than your body needs.

Obesity and Sleep Disorders

Obesity can have a pronounced impact on various sleep disorders, especially sleep apnea. In a vicious cycle, obesity leads to sleep apnea, and vice versa. Obesity is also a common denominator in various illnesses, including hypertension, asthma, diabetes, and heart disease. The economic impact, both directly and indirectly, of these conditions is tremendous.

So, what causes obesity?

As reported in many academic journals, the cause of obesity is multifactorial (meaning many factors come into play), including genetic and environmental causes. Poor quality of sleep and shorter duration of sleep both also show a direct correlation to obesity.

For overweight folks, I recommend a full panel blood test to rule out metabolic disorders. If they have a history of snoring and admit to being tired during the day, I order a sleep study to rule out sleep disorders like sleep apnea.

Thankfully, people with mild sleep apnea can often see a full resolution of their condition if they lose excess weight. For most of my clients, I recommend an initial weight loss goal of around 10% of their body weight.

Recently, federal and state government agencies have started to fund and promote research on the impact and treatment of obesity. It is my hope that some of this research will focus on how improving sleep hygiene is an integral step to combating obesity.

In the meantime, you can make a big difference in your daily routine by being mindful about the foods you eat at night and by decreasing the amount of time you watch TV or scroll on your phone or other handheld devices right before bed.

If you're having a hard time sleeping, it's tempting to stroll into the kitchen in your PJs and check the pantry for any satisfying midnight snacks. But as comforting as this ritual may be, it turns out that eating late actually hampers the natural sleeping process.

Eating a large quantity of food right before bed—even if it's healthy—activates your body's digestive system and signals that it's time to get active. So, as much as everyone loves a nighttime treat of cookies with milk, it's probably best to abstain from eating at this hour.

Of course, *when* you eat is just as important as *what* you eat. Eating too much fatty, spicy, or heavy food before bedtime can cause acid reflux and indigestion, interfering with our ability to stay asleep. So, if you're a more sensitive or light sleeper, avoiding these foods altogether at dinner may be in order.

How Else Does Eating Late at Night Affect Sleep?

So, how exactly does eating late at night make it hard to sleep? Beyond the physical discomfort of having a full stomach, the digestive process raises the body's internal temperature. This increase interferes with the natural drop in core temperature that helps you drift off to sleep at night.

In other words, sleep onset is triggered by a reduction of body temperature, and consuming food causes an *increase* in body temperature that can result in delayed sleep onset. The increased body temperature can also disrupt the body's circadian rhythm, delaying the secretion of melatonin, which is maximally secreted when your core body temperature drops. Without melatonin, it's much harder to fall asleep.

Folks who eat later or those who have a large meal prior to going to sleep have more episodes of waking up after falling asleep. A 2011 study found that any food eaten during the nocturnal period—including late dinners and bedtime snacks—interfered with getting a good night's sleep.[99] I recommend eating a small dinner: the earlier in the evening, the better.

Beyond this temporary problem, if eating at night becomes a habit, it's much more likely to lead to weight gain or even obesity. If a person does become obese, then this, in turn, creates even more sleep problems.

Obese folks are more likely to suffer from sleep apnea, which as we know, disrupts breathing, causes frequent awakenings, and overall makes it much more difficult to get a restful night of sleep. A 2019 study found that in people who already had sleep apnea, eating late at night made their symptoms worse.[100] Interestingly, the study also discovered that eating later for other meals, like breakfast and lunch, contributed to greater sleep latency and poor sleep quality.

Acid Reflux and Sleep

Spicy food, alcohol, and carbonated beverages are all well known to cause acid reflux (also known as heartburn). During the day, gravity and the lower esophageal sphincter (the valve that keeps the acid in the stomach) generally keeps the acid in the stomach where it belongs. When you're lying in bed at night, gravity no longer helps, plus the muscle tone of the esophageal sphincter is reduced in sleep, resulting in acid rushing back into the food passage. This, in turn, predisposes you to heartburn from gastric acid reflux.

When you have acid reflux, the discomfort of heartburn wakes you up. To make matters worse, these awakenings activate the sympathetic nervous system, resulting in increased heart rate and blood pressure.

To help with digestion, the stomach produces acid and enzymes whenever you consume food. But acid production in the stomach is at its peak between 2 and 4 a.m. This is also the time most awakenings from acid reflux happen.

Food tends to stay in the stomach between 40–120 minutes after you eat, so if you go to bed before the food has moved to your intestines, you're more at risk of acid reflux.

Heartburn affects as high as 40% of the US population at least once a month.[101] For most of us, acid reflux occurs occasionally as a result of something we've eaten. However, for some folks, acid reflux occurs regularly. This is called gastroesophageal reflux disease, or GERD.[102] Across the board, GERD compromises sleep quality.

A 2022 study showed that GERD led to a shorter overall sleep span and a decrease in sleep efficiency.[103] The more severe the symptoms of reflux are, the worse the quality of sleep.

Some people take antacids to relieve their symptoms, but unfortunately, your body still needs acid to be able to digest food. So taking these medications is not a great long-term solution. It's better to avoid heartburn-inducing foods and beverages foods altogether—or at least have them earlier in the day—*not* before bed.

Andrew

Andrew was a 50-year-old computer programmer who had severe GERD. He was also being treated for hypertension, diabetes, and obesity.

All day and often into the night, Andrew sat staring at a screen, typing. His diet had been high in carbohydrates, he ate a lot of fast food, and he loved energy drinks. Lately, he was working to eat a more gut-friendly diet to help relieve his gastrointestinal issues.

Andrew's family physician referred him to a gastroenterologist (a digestive system specialist) who performed an endoscopy (where they take a micro camera and look into his esophagus) to try to determine the cause of his condition.

Thankfully, there was no evidence of cancer, but the procedure showed that he had significant acid damage to his esophagus.

The gastroenterologist placed Andrew on an acid-suppressing medication, which helped partially. The doctor doubled his dose, and again, Andrew had some improvement. However, he wanted full relief from his GERD, so Andrew continued to push for a solution.

His primary care physician was aware of the correlation between severe GERD symptoms and the possibility of sleep apnea as a contributing factor. Sleep apnea can create negative pressure in the esophagus, which creates a suction effect, pulling the acid up the esophagus.

The physician referred Andrew to me, and I set him up with a home sleep study. Again, not unexpectedly given his medical history, the study showed severe sleep apnea.

He was prescribed a CPAP machine, and this made a significant difference. Andrew also consulted with a dietitian and changed his food habits, having his evening meals earlier and avoiding fatty and acidic foods.

After six months, he was weaned off his acid-suppressing medication, and he had also lost 40 pounds in the process. He continues to use his CPAP machine. Eventually, Andrew was doing so well that I was able to lower the pressure on his CPAP machine. He continues to do well to this day.

Obesity and Medical Issues

It seems obvious that reduction in sleep time and quality can contribute to obesity. Obesity, in turn, makes it harder to sleep and is a leading cause of OSA, which can have a significant impact on various medical conditions. It is a vicious cycle, as obesity is also a common denominator for other illnesses, including hypertension, diabetes, heart disease and osteoarthritis, all of which can make sleep more difficult.[104]

Eating Right for Great Sleep

Meal timing isn't the only thing that matters when it comes to getting a good night's sleep. Choosing the *right* foods also plays a part. We already know that caffeine, alcohol, high-fat, and high-acid foods are a bad idea close to bedtime. However, most people don't realize that even if they eat relatively healthy foods with lots of protein at night, it can make it difficult to sleep because proteins require so much energy to digest.

So, what should we be eating to get better quality sleep?

Instead of junk food, reach for high-fiber foods like fruits and vegetables, as well as complex carbohydrates like whole wheat bread or brown rice. These foods are easy to digest and don't cause a sugar crash like other simple carbs. Veggies and complex carbs are smart choices to make all day long, but especially when you're preparing for bed.[105]

Digestion naturally slows down at night, so choose something that's easy to digest but will keep you satisfied until morning.

Eating a healthy diet and getting good quality sleep are two of the best measures you can take to protect your health. Luckily, these two things serve each other. If you're getting plenty of sleep, you're more likely to reach for nutrient-dense foods and eat moderate portion sizes. In turn, if you're eating well, your body is more likely to fall asleep quickly and stay asleep throughout the night.

If one of these functions starts to derail—for instance, if you lose sleep because of work stress or eat poorly because you're on vacation—then it's easy for the other to get off track as well. For that reason, it's essential to course-correct after any disrupting event, so that your body can return to equilibrium.

When you're eating right, great sleep should follow.

Chapter 7

Sleep and Sexual Health

Nathan came to see me to be evaluated for sleep apnea, and as we sat down in my office, I could tell he was struggling with embarrassment.

I asked him about his family, and he told me his wife, Hannah, was still "drop dead gorgeous" even after having two kids, and she was an amazing cook. (It was obvious that he enjoyed her cooking!)

He was only 45 years old, but he had a history of high blood pressure and diabetes (he said blood pressure issues ran in his family). He hadn't been sleeping well, though, and Hannah had been complaining that his snoring was super loud and was keeping her awake.

As we continued to talk, he shared how difficult things were in the bedroom. His primary care physician had done a physical examination and full panel blood test that showed while Nathan's testosterone level was lower than most men of his age, there were no others evident causes of his erectile dysfunction (ED).

I spent some time talking with him about how sleep issues (including sleep apnea) can impact sexual health and reassured him that he was far from unusual. I told him that, sadly, many men suffer in silence and commended him on seeking help.

I wasn't at all surprised when his home sleep study showed severe sleep apnea.

I prescribed CPAP treatment, and I also told him that to get his blood pressure and diabetes under control, a fitness program could be a huge benefit.

Six months later, when Nathan came in for his follow-up appointment, he told me he had not only *joined* the local gym, but he was also actually *going*. . . and enjoying it.

He also said his libido had improved, and his blood work showed his testosterone levels had returned to normal. The combination of his CPAP and weight loss had also greatly improved his diabetes and blood pressure. So, he was not only feeling better, but he was also looking better and feeling better about himself overall.

And although he said using a CPAP wasn't the sexiest, he knew it was worth it to feel healthier and get back to enjoying intimacy with his wife.

☽

Pop songs often celebrate the joy of staying up all night to have sex. Like Daft Punk's 2013 hit, "Get Lucky," songwriters are seemingly thrilled to lose a night of sleep to enjoy more intercourse. However, research suggests that people who don't get enough sleep are often having *less* sex. That's because getting adequate sleep nourishes our sexual health, while skimping on shuteye puts it at risk.

Sex and sleep, just like sleep and other areas of health, share a bidirectional relationship. When we sleep better, we are able to enjoy having sex, and when we have sex, we're more likely to sleep better. That's because sex releases hormones like prolactin and oxytocin.[106]

Oxytocin is commonly known as the "love hormone" as it creates a feeling of pleasantness, connection, and relaxation. As a result, many people report being able to sleep better after sex since oxytocin relaxes us and makes it easier to sleep.

Prolactin, also released during intercourse, fosters relaxation, and it makes it easier to drift off to sleep. (As the name suggests, it's also responsible for the creation of breast milk.)

When sex isn't occurring, these hormones aren't released, making it more difficult for some people to sleep. And when sleep isn't happening, sex becomes less appealing. People who are sleep-deprived tend to have a lower libido and an increased risk of sexual dysfunction.

This occurs partly because insomnia creates stress, which causes the brain to decrease its production of sex hormones and increase its production of stress hormones. Not only that, but sleep-deprived individuals may simply be *too tired* to have sex.

While lack of sleep is unavoidable in some phases of life—like while caring for a newborn or studying for exams—I recommend that people should try to get as much sleep as possible. If sleep deprivation outlasts the original precipitating factor, it's generally time to talk to your doctor about underlying sleep issues before they start hampering your sex life.

Sexual Dysfunction in Men

Sexual function in men typically boils down to one thing: their ability to achieve and maintain an erection. Other symptoms, like low libido, loss of body hair, and ejaculation issues (either ejaculating too soon, too late, or not at all) are included when we discuss men's sexual dysfunction, although they're not as primary as erection. ED is the most primary form of male sexual dysfunction.

Previously, ED was considered part of the natural aging process. While it's true that ED is certainly more common in middle and later life, aging isn't always the main culprit. Often, ED is linked to another problem like heart disease, obesity, diabetes, high cholesterol, high blood pressure, or sleep apnea.[107] Sometimes, ED is a side effect of certain medications. These can include antidepressants, antiandrogens, tranquilizers, sedatives, and appetite suppressants.

Lifestyle choices can also contribute to ED, including smoking, drinking, and not getting sufficient exercise. Emotional distress or mental illness can also contribute to ED.

Since there can be several different causes for ED, I recommend that patients are screened for other disorders before writing it off as just a natural part of the aging process.

About 52% of men report some form of ED in their lives.[108] Naturally, the rate is lower among younger men. However, doctors estimate that this number is much higher in real life.

According to a study done in 2003, of 500 men who saw a urologist for another issue, 44% experienced ED but never spoke about it with their doctor. The reasons for staying silent varied. Some reported that they considered it a natural side effect of aging, and therefore, it wasn't worth treating. Others claimed they didn't know that ED fell within the purview of urologists. But the most common reason was embarrassment. In fact, 74% of these men were simply too embarrassed to mention this problem to their urologist, even though urologists can treat this problem.[109]

Erectile Dysfunction's Impact on Quality of Life

Unfortunately, ED affects more than just sexual satisfaction. A recent study by PubMed gathered findings from 20 different studies regarding ED's effect on quality of life. The results were alarming. Men with ED reported a significantly lower quality of life than their peers without ED. Beyond that, folks with ED struggled more economically. They were more likely to miss work and when they did show up, they had lower productivity metrics than their coworkers without ED.[110]

In addition, ED tends to hinder men's relationships with their partners. In heterosexual relationships, women whose partners had ED reported less satisfaction with their sex lives. Many of them reported that they considered ED a problem in their relationship. In one Swedish study, 82% of women whose partners had ED reported that they were sexually dissatisfied.[111]

Low Libido

Poor sexual function and low libido are more prevalent in people who have sleep apnea. Studies have shown that when compared to people without sleep apnea, men with OSA attempt sex less often, usually due to fatigue.[112]

While the exact relationship between OSA and sexual dysfunction is not understood, experts believe it's related to fatigue and the lack of oxygen caused by apnea. People with untreated sleep apnea tend to complain of being tired all the time, which is one factor that leads to low libido, making them less interested in sex.

Also, the resultant hypoxia (lower oxygen) associated with sleep apnea affects the neural process of an erection. The erection phenomenon is both a vascular *and* a neural event. When stimulated, the nerves increase energy to the penis and the heart circulates more blood to this area, causing the erection. When sleep apnea intermittently deprives both the neural and vascular systems of oxygen during the night, erection becomes more difficult.

Aside from simply affecting the mechanics of an erection, sleep apnea also causes an overall decrease in testosterone production. This also inhibits the sex drive and makes erections more difficult to achieve.

In a study of over 1,000 men with ED, 91% of them had at least mild sleep apnea.[113] And with those with severe sleep apnea, there was a notable decrease in nitric oxide (the chemical that improves blood flow) production in folks.

Nitric oxide dilates the blood vessels, and so if there isn't enough of it in the system, the vasodilatory (expansion of blood vessel) process that is needed for an erection won't occur. In other words, the blood vessels shrink instead of expanding. All these different studies confirm one thing—that ED is complex and is frequently related to sleep issues.

Sex Hormone Irregularities in People with Sleep Apnea

In the medical community, it's common knowledge that reduced sleep time is associated with lower testosterone levels. Insufficient sleep disrupts the brain–sex organ regulation (hypothalamic-pituitary-gonadal) in both men and women.

Unfortunately, in modern society, there are many other causes for low testosterone and high estrogen. Certain foods like red kidney beans, excess red meat, processed foods, and excess alcohol also contribute to increased estrogen, plus many of the everyday toiletries we use contain a sealant that can increase estrogen levels.[114]

In my own research, I've found that some coffee pods, lip balm, deodorant, and cologne all contain estrogen. Higher levels of estrogen affect testosterone, as it binds to the protein molecules competitively, thus lowering the levels of free testosterone in the blood.

And a lack of testosterone can predispose men to sleep apnea due to the increased upper airway collapsibility (oropharyngeal collapse).

Sleep-Related Sexual Dysfunction in Women

While scientists typically measure men's sexual health by the ability to have an erection, women's sexuality is more nuanced as it is more difficult to quantify than men's; therefore, it has often been overlooked by researchers.

However, researchers are beginning to shine the spotlight on how sleep—and lack of sleep—impacts women's sexual health.

For instance, a 2015 study found that "longer sleep duration was related to greater next-day sexual desire, and that a one-hour increase in sleep length corresponded to a 14% increase in odds of engaging in partnered sexual activity." This study measured women's sexual health by sexual desire, "subjective arousal," and "orgasmic functioning." [115]

These results are especially promising since the study showed that even a relatively minor increase in the amount of sleep obtained created significant rewards.

Another study found that women with poor sleep quality were 48% more likely to report female sexual dysfunction than women with good sleep quality. The same study also reported that women who were sexually active were more likely to enjoy high-quality sleep than women who were not currently sexually active.[116] This may be a result of the relaxing hormones that are released after sex, like oxytocin and prolactin.

Aside from a general lack of sleep, women with OSA, in particular, are also at a higher risk of developing sexual difficulties. In one study, a diagnosis of sleep apnea alone—regardless of how mild—was enough to put women at risk for sexual dysfunction. The severity of the sleep apnea didn't seem to play a role in how severe the sexual difficulties were.[117]

Sleep Disorders and Their Effect on Fertility

Not surprisingly, there's a direct correlation between sex and fertility. When sexual function is compromised due to lack of sleep, fertility may be affected as well. In men, sleep duration of 6.5 hours is associated with a decrease in semen volume and total sperm count, compared to men who slept longer.[118]

While most research has focused on men, scientists have identified a link between chronic sleeplessness and lower fertility in women. There are many theories for why this may occur. Many scientists believe that insomnia activates the hypothalamic-pituitary-adrenal axis, which triggers the release of stress hormones.[119]

There is also a strong relationship between sleep apnea and polycystic ovary syndrome, a disorder seen in women of reproductive age group associated with obesity, insulin resistance, and fluid filled sacs (cysts) in the ovaries, infertility, and increased levels of testosterone. In fact, one study found that obstructive sleep apnea was present in 35% of obese women with this syndrome.[120]

A 2013 study focused on infertile women who were undergoing intrauterine insemination treatment to try to become pregnant. Intrauterine insemination is a treatment in which a doctor directly inserts the sperm into the uterus, as this increases the likelihood of conception as compared to intercourse. The study found that of the women they studied who were all struggling with infertility, about 35% also reported sleep disturbances.[121]

The Effects of CPAP Treatment and How It Improves Sexual Health

A CPAP machine does not *look* sexy, but if you sleep better, you might *feel* sexy!

As devastating as sleep apnea can be to sexual health, hope is available in the form of CPAP therapy. Use of a CPAP machine is linked to notable improvement of sexual functioning in people with sleep apnea. Even more encouraging, when using a CPAP machine to manage their sleep apnea, many see relief of their other health disorders as well.

In one study conducted by Walter Reed National Military Medical Center, researchers found that CPAP therapy improved mild ED in 50% of participants. In people with severe ED, 27% of them reported better sexual function.[122]

Interestingly, CPAP seems to also improve sexual function for women with sleep apnea. In a 2018 study, women who used a CPAP machine every night for a year reported a one- to two-point improvement in their libido.[123]

While some people are hesitant to start CPAP therapy because they're worried it will make their sex life worse (largely due to worries that the contraption looks incredibly unsexy while in use), the opposite has proven to be true.

Even though the machine and mask themselves may not be the most appealing nighttime accessories, the overall health benefits are worth it. Making the flow of oxygen more consistent throughout the night relieves a host of health problems, boosts energy, and increases libido and sexual performance.

Testosterone deficiency in men is associated with OSA, and testosterone replacement treatment can cause or worsen OSA.[124] It is highly recommended that administration of such hormones and medications be handled by physicians with significant expertise in this specialty.

As we've established, sleep is essential for all aspects of health. This is just as true for sexual health as it is for more commonly discussed functions. For some people, improving their sex life can be as simple as implementing better sleep strategies.

For others, some treatment may be required to help them get back on track with their sleeping—and subsequently, with their sex life as well. Fostering health in this sometimes-overlooked field is essential, since sex has such a huge impact on quality of life and relationships.

Sexual relationships are important component of happiness in couple's life and getting treatment for conditions like insomnia, sleep apnea, depression, menopause, environmental sleep disorder (snoring) that affect sleep quality and duration can result in us living happier lives.[125]

Chapter 8

Sleep and Children

Benjamin was a precocious 10-year-old recently diagnosed with ADHD. He loved Mandalorian Legos, dinosaurs, and Minecraft, and he had lots of friends who lived on his cul-de-sac.

I had given a talk at a local conference on the importance of sleep in children, and his mom, Lela, was in attendance. After my talk, she immediately called my office to make an appointment. Benjamin did not have any developmental issues, and all his milestones seemed normal. However, Lela mentioned that her son exhibited mild snoring.

A few minutes into our conversation, she also mentioned he had been more withdrawn recently and had stopped going to sleepovers. After a bit more discussion, Benjamin admitted that he'd been wetting the bed and was afraid that this could happen at his friends' homes.

Benjamin's clinical exam was normal except for moderately enlarged tonsils. The sleep study revealed that Benjamin did, in fact, have sleep apnea, and I referred him to an ear, nose, and throat surgeon who removed his tonsils and adenoids.

When I saw Benjamin for a follow-up visit, his bedwetting had resolved, and his behavior and concentration had also improved. He was no longer afraid of spending nights with his friends.

It felt like a sheer coincidence that Lela had attended the conference and learned about the correlation between bedwetting, ADHD, and sleep apnea. Otherwise, her son's symptoms of sleep apnea could have continued to be misdiagnosed simply as ADHD, and his snoring would not have been resolved.

The Developmental Nature of Sleep

One day, a nine-year-old child approached me and asked, "Doctor John, can I ask you a question?"

"Sure, buddy."

"I have a baby sister who sleeps all the time. She's six months old. I'm worried she's never going to get taller because she's always sleeping!"

"Hmm. . . I understand your concern. But the truth is, sleeping is what's going to help her grow the most."

☽

Sleep is essential for children's overall growth, development, and well-being. Here are a few reasons why children need sufficient sleep:

Physical growth: Sleep plays a crucial role in supporting physical growth and development in children. During sleep, the body releases growth hormones that help with the growth of bones and organs, muscle development, and tissue repair.

Cognitive development: Sleep is closely linked to cognitive processes such as memory consolidation, learning, and problem-solving. Sufficient sleep allows children's brains to process and store information effectively, facilitating optimal cognitive development.

Emotional regulation: Adequate sleep helps stabilize mood, reduce irritability, and promote emotional well-being in children, so a well-rested child is better equipped to regulate their emotions and handle daily stressors.

Immune function: Sleep plays a vital role in strengthening the immune system, which helps protect children from illnesses. During sleep, the body activates immune cells and proteins that combat infections and support overall immune function.

Behavior and attention: Insufficient sleep can negatively impact children's behavior and attention span. Sleep deprivation may contribute to irritability, hyperactivity, impulsiveness, and difficulties with concentration and learning.

Physical health: Adequate sleep is linked to a lower risk of obesity as it influences hunger-regulating hormones and helps maintain a healthy metabolism. Additionally, proper sleep supports cardiovascular health and reduces the risk of chronic conditions later in life.

The amount of sleep children need varies with age. Newborns and infants require the most sleep, typically between 14 and 18 hours per day. As children grow, the recommended sleep duration gradually decreases, but they still need significant amounts of sleep. Preschoolers (3–5 years) typically require 10–13 hours, school-age children (6–13 years) need 9–11 hours, and teenagers (14–17 years) benefit from 8–10 hours of sleep each night.[126]

It is important for parents and caregivers to establish consistent sleep routines and create a conducive sleep environment to ensure children get the sleep they need for their optimal growth, development, and overall well-being.

Children's bodies secrete HGH (human growth hormone) while they're asleep, which is part of the reason younger children and babies need so many hours of rest in a day. It helps ensure that they reach their full growth potential.

Sleep disorders are common in children. At least 25–50% of children will experience some sleep-related issue during their childhood.[127] This can have a profound impact on a child's mood, academic performance, and overall well-being.

However, if we can identify the problem early and develop a treatment plan, we can usually fully reverse the issue. Common sleep disorders in children are behavioral insomnia, night terrors and nightmares, sleep apnea, sleepwalking, delayed sleep phase, and restless leg syndrome.

General Insomnia in Children

By nature, children are sound sleepers; they usually don't have the worries of the world on their shoulders. They are active, play hard, and are usually exhausted after a long day of school, so they fall asleep in an instant.

But sadly, the incidence of insomnia is roughly 20–30% in children and adolescents, according to research in 2020.[128]

I suspect the incidence is even higher now due to things like increased screen time and how kids are more aware of changing social constructs.

Emma

Emma was a quiet 11-year-old girl with big brown eyes who had been having difficulty sleeping for the six months leading up to our meeting. Emma's stepmom admitted that Emma's behavioral and sleep issues started after her parents' bitter divorce and custody battle.

Other than that, Emma was a healthy child who had good grades and was active in sports (she was a goalie on her soccer team). There were no symptoms of restless legs or sleep apnea, and she was usually in bed by 9 p.m.

When Emma and I chatted and I asked her why she couldn't sleep, she mentioned that she's been having difficulty adjusting to her new family (living with her dad, his new wife, and her new step siblings). Plus, there had been a deadly school shooting near where she lived.

Emma had an iPad she used for school, and since she had many questions about the shooting, she spent many hours in her bedroom at night, reading about what had happened and watching media coverage of the event. This left her confused and anxious.

She had two things working against her: the increased screen time at night had led to insufficient sleep, and the complex subject for her age had left her anxious, which then worsened her sleep.

I arranged a meeting with a psychologist and family therapist to help her try to better understand this complex and delicate issue. Some of these sessions also included her parents and stepparents. They all agreed she wasn't allowed to go to sleep with her iPad.

When I saw Emma for a follow-up visit, she was coping better, and her sleep quality had improved significantly.

☾

Most causes of insomnia are behaviorally induced, but there are several other reasons for insomnia in kids. These include medical conditions such as asthma, eczema, pain from sports and related injuries, seasonal allergies, and headaches. Children who are suffering from depression and anxiety also have a significantly higher incidence of insomnia.

Insomnia and sleep-related complaints are some of the most common reasons for visits to the pediatrician's office.[129] In fact, incidences of insomnia can be as high as 80% in children with cognitive disabilities and other associated syndromes, like Down syndrome.[130]

In fact, younger children who get less than the recommended amount of sleep also struggle in virtually all spheres of life. Insufficient sleep in this age group is associated with behavioral, cognitive and mood changes.[131]

A study conducted by the University of Maryland surveyed 4,000 children between the ages of 9 and 10 where those who had nine more hours of sleep were compared to children of the same age who slept less than nine hours. The study revealed that *the children who had less sleep had more mental and behavioral issues*. Less sleep was also linked to increased stress, anxiety, depression, and aggressive behavior.[132]

Another study found that children between ages 3 and 7 who didn't get enough sleep also had issues with emotional control and peer relationships.[133] For children and teens who are already suffering from anxiety and depression, poor and insufficient sleep exacerbate their symptoms. Unfortunately, these negative outcomes don't seem to resolve over time unless sleep problems are corrected. For this reason, it's crucial that parents and caregivers intervene early to undo some of the detrimental effects of sleep deprivation.[134]

Aside from poor sleep routines and having an irregular bedtime, there are several other sleep disorders that can cause poor sleep or full-blown insomnia in children.

As we discussed in an earlier chapter, anxiety, depression, and mood disorders can also hinder sleep in children, resulting in insomnia. In children and teens with insomnia, I always recommend screening for mental health disorders before I start treatment, as these can create a vicious cycle. Poor sleep worsens mental health, and vice versa.

Insomnia can be a cry for help in young children who are battling depression and anxiety, but don't yet have the vocabulary to express how they feel. Children who are victims of abuse also have a significantly higher incidence of insomnia.

As caregivers, we need to be vigilant about uncovering why a child is not sleeping enough. By identifying and addressing the underlying reasons—whether it is simply too much screen time or an actual medical or mental health condition—we can help children restore quality of sleep. Helping our children get the recommended amount of high-quality sleep will pay dividends as our children grow, since sleep is essential for physical, academic, social, and emotional well-being.

Sleepwalking

Sleepwalking (somnambulism) is a very common phenomenon in children, with up to 10–15% of children (or more accurately, their caregivers) reporting some episode of sleepwalking. Children have a relatively higher percentage of deep sleep (stage 3 of non-REM sleep), which makes them slightly more prone to sleepwalking.

In this deep sleep state, the mind and body can still function, so children are still able to walk, unlike in REM sleep, in which the muscles are paralyzed. Sleepwalking episodes most often happen in the first third of the night, as the density of deep sleep is highest at that time.

Episodes normally last from a few seconds to a few minutes. Children are totally unaware of the episodes while they are happening, and they usually have no recollection when they wake up. Sleepwalking is a self-limiting disorder, which means it typically resolves without treatment. This usually happens when the child ages and the density of slow-wave sleep is reduced. Sleepwalking typically peaks between ages 6 and 8, and it usually resolves before teenage years.

If your child has sleepwalking episodes, it's important to ensure their safety. This means making sure there are no dangerous objects in the child's room and that the bed is relatively low to the ground. It's also better if their bedroom is on a lower floor of the house to reduce the risk of falling out of windows or down any stairs. Doors and windows should be closed, and if the child is sleeping on a higher floor, there should be a gate at the stairs.

Though sleepwalking can occur sporadically, there are triggers which make it more likely. Sleep deprivation and insufficient sleep are the usual culprits. For this reason, it is imperative that children maintain a strict sleep schedule that guarantees them at least 9–11 hours (depending on the child's age) a night.

If your child's sleepwalking becomes a problem, please consult with a pediatrician or a sleep specialist to rule out other sleep disorders or underlying factors that could be a contributing factor.

Night Terrors and Nightmares

There's nothing quite like being awoken in the middle of the night to the sound of your child's screaming with a night terror. And "terror" is a good way to describe it.

Night terrors are characterized by sudden, frightful awakenings that occur in the first third of the night, usually during the first 3–4 hours after sleep onset. The child can wake up crying, thrashing around, or sitting upright in bed. Usually, the dreams cannot be recollected, and the child appears confused, not remembering what made them so upset. Children can be reassured and put back to sleep after the episode. (As parents, it might not be as easy to go back to sleep. . .)

Nightmares are different. They occur during REM sleep, typically toward the later part of the night. The child often wakes up during a nightmare, scared and upset. It is not unusual for them to remember the nightmare.

If night terrors or nightmares tend to happen at a set time of the night, a parent can enter the bedroom a few minutes prior to the usual onset time and gently speak to the child, call their name, and help them change their sleeping position. If this technique is followed for a few weeks, the symptoms usually subside.

Parents also need to make sure the bedroom is safe and good sleep routines are maintained, meaning regular bedtime, reducing screen time, and avoiding heavy meals before bed.

These disorders can be inherited and usually peak at age 3–6. Most children outgrow them by 8–12 years of age.

Bedwetting

Bedwetting is another common childhood disorder which should resolve naturally by ages 6–8. Bedwetting could also be hereditary. In some children, the bladder is simply not fully developed by the time they stop wearing diapers.

Bedwetting can be embarrassing to children, especially if they attend sleepovers. For most children, limiting fluid intake closer to bedtime could be helpful. If the bedwetting pattern continues even after fluids are limited, parents may want to implement an alarm so the child can be awakened and use the restroom at a designated time.

If this is still an issue by age 10, then a visit to a pediatrician or sleep specialist is recommended to investigate other causes. Bedwetting could also be a sign of stress, urinary tract infections, diabetes, or sleep apnea, as described in Benjamin's story.

Childhood Behavioral Insomnia

Behavioral insomnia is the most common sleep disorder among children. I call it a 50/50 problem, where the blame is partly on the child and partly on the parents who often give in, creating a negative reinforcement cycle. Often, parents think they are doing their children a favor by succumbing to their requests to stay up later. However, it's easy for codependency to take hold when the child takes control of the parent-child relationship and their *wants* become *demands*.

Children often try to manipulate the more lenient parent, which can result in discord between the two parents. This type of behavior can result in poor quality of sleep for all parties involved.

Like most children, my son was a master manipulator when it came to bedtime. (This was before I became a sleep specialist.) When Brandon was around three years old, we had to listen to his singing, tell him a story, listen to *his* story, tell another story, and on and on. Finally, he would fall asleep an hour later, holding onto my wife's hair.

After my fellowship in sleep medicine, I realized there was an easy fix. My wife, Dotty, and I needed to stand our ground and stop giving in to Brandon's countless pre-bedtime needs. We let him know he would get one bedtime story, and that was that. He had to go to sleep by himself.

The first week was difficult, as he resisted this new boundary with loud screaming and wailing, but by the eighth night, it was much better, and after that, it became a habit. It was a long week but, ultimately, the best for all of us.

Instilling a healthy sleeping ritual for Rachael, our second-born child, was easy as we already knew what to do and what *not* to do.

Two Types of Behavioral Insomnia in Children

There are two main types of behavioral insomnia in children: Sleep-onset association, and limit-setting insomnia.

In sleep-onset association insomnia, the child needs the parent's help to rock or feed them to sleep. The child associates the onset of sleep with an action by the parent, and they lose the ability to go to sleep by their own means.

In limit-setting insomnia, the child has several demands prior to going to sleep. This is what was happening with my first child. It may start out with good intentions by the parents, but then it shifts, and the parents tend to cave under pressure and carry out their child's requests—or more accurately, *demands*—and this reinforces the behavior.

This disorder can be compounded by a bedtime that is too early, and by parents who often succumb to the whims of their children. Although, sometimes, it's easier said than done, the solution is not very complicated: keep the bedtime routine simple and have a fixed schedule.

Additionally, children need to know that they can, and should, go to sleep by themselves. Reading a relaxing book (a hard copy, *not* on any devices) before bedtime could be a good nighttime ritual. And avoiding TV time, social media, and video games close to bedtime can be very helpful.

In my experience, adding a positive reinforcement also helps, such as giving a reward at the end of the week for consistently going to bed on their own. It can be tough at first, but a little bit of effort will do the whole family a world of good in the long run. The key is both parents working together and being consistent with the bedtime rules.

Restless Legs Syndrome

Restless legs syndrome is a condition that causes a child an uncomfortable urge to move their legs. This urge to move usually happens in the evening or at bedtime, but it can also occur at other times when the child's legs have been inactive, such as when they have been sitting still for a long time (e.g., during long car rides or while watching a movie).

To get relief, the child usually ends up stretching or moving their legs. Sometimes they have to toss and turn or get up and walk to get relief. RLS can affect sleep onset, resulting in reduction in total sleep time and daytime sleepiness the next day.

In the US, approximately 1.5 million children and adolescents are estimated to have RLS, and over a third of them report symptoms before 20 years of age.[135]

The most common causes are deficiencies in iron (especially ferritin), vitamin B12, folate, and magnesium.[136] RLS usually runs in the family,[137] and there is also a racial predisposition, with Caucasians suffering at a much higher rate.[138]

Globally, the incidence of RLS in children varies widely.[139] The exact cause is unknown; however, there are several medications—especially antidepressants and antihistamines—that can *cause* RLS as a side effect.

Good sleep routines, avoidance of caffeine products, gentle exercises, and muscle relaxation techniques, such as stretching and repetitive movements, are recommended. I also recommend checking the child's medications, especially over-the-counter medications like antihistamines, which could be the culprit.

If the child's symptoms continue after good sleep strategies are introduced, I typically check their iron, ferritin, vitamin B12, folate, and magnesium levels. If any of these levels are low, I recommend adding a supplement, especially if the tests reveal low iron.

The enzyme that is responsible for making dopamine in the part of the brain that controls movements is iron-dependent. Hence, adding an iron supplement is often the first step in management of RLS.

Typically, when these steps are taken, symptoms improve dramatically. In-lab sleep studies are rarely needed, except in situations when other sleep disorders are suspected.

Obstructive Sleep Apnea in Children

Sleep apnea is most common in adults, but children can also be affected. The difference is that the symptoms are often subtle in children. Symptoms in children may include the following:

- Sub-par performance in school due to chronic sleepiness, exhaustion, and poor focus
- Sweating during sleep, as the heart and lungs are working harder to bring air into the body

- Snoring with an inward rib movement because the lungs are trying to get more oxygen into the body
- Learning and behavior issues, often diagnosed as ADHD
- Sluggishness or sleepiness, often misinterpreted as laziness in the classroom
- Odd sleeping positions
- Bedwetting

If your child shows any of these symptoms, it's worth having them evaluated by a pediatrician or a sleep specialist to rule out sleep apnea. It's also a good idea to get your child's sleep examined if they've been diagnosed with ADHD, since poor sleep due to sleep apnea could be one of the root causes of attention and behavioral problems.

A hospital sleep study (in-lab, attended sleep study) is needed to diagnose pediatric sleep apnea. In children with sleep apnea, the main cause of obstruction is usually enlarged tonsils and adenoids. Therefore, a tonsillectomy and adenoidectomy help resolve the issue. However, some children may need CPAP therapy, decongestion medication, or a steroid nasal spray.

Both my children had symptoms of sleep apnea. My son, who was eight at the time, was exhausted when he woke up in the morning—even after sleeping 10 hours the night before. He would fall back to sleep on his way to school. He also snored loudly at night. My daughter, who was seven, didn't snore much, but she had frequent upper airway respiratory infections. We had a call from the school that she was sleeping in her classes and her grades were falling.

After taking them to the pediatrician, it was determined that they both had enlarged tonsils and adenoids and they both ended up having their tonsils and adenoids removed. The surgeries were a success and they had significant improvements—my wife and I both thought it was a pretty dramatic change! They didn't have any more symptoms after that (well, that is until college, when they were burning the candle at both ends, as the saying goes).

Sleep Apnea and Cognitive Impairment in Children

In younger children, ages 3–5, OSA (obstructive sleep apnea, as you may recall) tends to create more behavioral than cognitive problems. Symptoms often include poor attention span and impaired executive functioning.

For older children, cognitive issues are also present. Children aged 6–12 showed deficits in "visuo-spatial memory, attention, and working memory."[140]

OSA also diminished the children's *phonological* processing, which is the process needed for children to learn how to read. A 2014 study showed that OSA may even affect a child's ability to feel empathy.[141] Children diagnosed with ADHD could have untreated OSA, which could mean the cause of their symptoms is from a lack of restful sleep due to repeated awakenings during the night.

Despite these concerning results, there is evidence that treating OSA early can help prevent cognitive deficits from becoming permanent. Children who have had tonsillectomy and adenoidectomy surgery earlier for treating sleep apnea tend to fair better on cognitive assessments, suggesting that treating OSA as early as possible can protect against poor cognitive outcomes. Thus, early diagnosis and treatment is recommended.

Sleep and School Performance

If you think back to your high school or college days, you can probably remember pulling at least one all-nighter to prepare for a test. These nights typically involve lots of snacks, energy drinks, and perhaps copious amounts of flash cards scattered around. The unfortunate thing is that cramming doesn't really work.

That's because sleep—not flashcards—is the most important part of learning and memory-making. Nighttime is when our brains store and consolidate what we've learned so we can access it later. For these reasons, skipping out on sleep and staying up late and studying to perform better on a test is a fool's errand.

Adequate sleep is essential for all aspects of learning, especially in children. They need the most sleep of any age because their bodies are growing so quickly, and because their main job at this stage of life is to learn as much as possible. Not only does lack of sleep compromise our ability to store information, but it also makes it hard to muster the concentration required to learn new things in the first place.

Unfortunately, a study done in 2013 shows that many children are not getting the sleep they need. This lack of sleep can significantly compromise their ability to pay attention and synthesize knowledge, causing their academic performance to suffer.[142]

How Much Sleep Are Children Getting?

According to a study conducted between 2016 and 2018, 34.9% of children between the ages of four months and 17 years are getting less sleep than the recommended amount for their age.[143]

Remember, as I stated at the beginning of this chapter,

- newborns and infants typically require between 14 and 18 hours of sleep per day,
- preschoolers (3–5 years) typically require 10–13 hours,
- school-age children (6–13 years) need 9–11 hours,
- and teenagers (14–17 years) benefit from 8–10 hours of sleep each night.

A CDC study relied on parents to answer questions about their children's sleep habits and the amount of time they slept on average.[144] Unsurprisingly, the children who had regular bedtimes tended to get more sleep than their counterparts who didn't. Children whose parents reported lower income levels also tended to report shorter sleep times for their children, likely due to their parents' shift work or more noisy sleeping environments.[145]

The problem of insufficient sleep seems to only get worse as children get older. One study found that among middle school students, six out of 10 did not get the amount of sleep needed. For high school students, that number rose to seven out of 10. A larger analysis evaluating over 40 studies revealed that daily sleep time during the week was seven hours and 40 minutes among teenagers; this amount is consistent with a diagnosis of insufficient sleep.[146]

As teens require 8–10 hours of sleep. That said, even this small differential was enough to cause significant sleepiness and academic impairment in the study participants. I like to tell my clients that while there's only a 20-minute difference between seven hours and 40 minutes and eight hours, *every minute counts*. It's like having 99 cents versus a whole dollar.

Additionally, children fall on both sides of this range, meaning some of the teenagers getting 7 hours and 40 minutes might *need* 10 hours, meaning they're operating at a two-hour and 20-minute loss every day.

Children, Sleep, and Mental Health

Unfortunately, with the advent of social media, many children are sleep-deprived, losing an average of eight hours of sleep each week—*one entire night of sleep.*[147] It is especially important for children and young adults to have the *optimal* amount of sleep to ensure emotional well-being.

On average, children as young as eight years old spend at least three hours—at times longer—a day on social media and compromise on the duration of sleep they get, simply so they can spend more time on their apps.[148] As a result, many are diagnosed with insomnia. And since they cannot sleep well, they become anxious.

This feeds into the negative cycle of anxiety worsening their sleep, even resulting in depression. Poor sleep can also interfere with learning and academic achievements.

Melatonin and Kids

Over the past few years, more and more folks have started purchasing melatonin as an over-the-counter sleep aid, including for their children.[149]

Melatonin is a chemical that the body produces to induce sleep. So, is it better to add *more* to help the body drift off more easily? As a sleep doctor, I have several concerns about this trend, and *I do not recommend melatonin for children.*

First, relying on melatonin as a sleep aid in the long-term can undermine your body's natural ability to fall asleep.

Second, children should naturally be sound sleepers. If your child requires medicine to fall asleep on a regular basis, it's worth looking at their sleep hygiene or having them evaluated for other causes.

Third, according to a recent article from *Harvard Health Publishing*, melatonin is not regulated by the FDA, meaning that doses can vary from pill to pill, with the most variability in chewable tablets—the product most commonly given to children.[150]

As a parent, I understand wanting to get your child to sleep without a fight. However, *medications should be a last resort* and should only be used after you've consulted with your pediatrician, even if the drug you're giving your child is purchased over the counter.

Melatonin does not put you to sleep; it can only change the time when you go sleep, hence I use it only for clock issues like advanced sleep phase syndrome (ASPS), delayed sleep phase syndrome (DSPS), and jet lag.

Here's when to seek help: If your child has behavioral and learning difficulties, if they snore, if they sleep less than eight hours, or if they feel tired despite sleeping more than 10 hours, make sure their pediatrician looks into their sleep habits.

Finally: Wondering about the benefit of naps? We'll address that in Chapter 12 (Sleep, Performance, and Success).

Chapter 9

Sleep and Teens

Kayla was a bright 15-year-old girl who was brought to the office by her parents because they had noticed her grades were slipping, and she was irritable and fighting with her siblings much more frequently (*way* more than normal).

Her teachers were also expressing concern over Kayla being less attentive in class. She had been a straight-A student who was enthusiastic and eager to learn just a few months ago, but by the time I met her, she was less interested in class.

Her mom knew Kayla hadn't been sleeping well and often raided the kitchen late at night. She also said she was practically dragging Kayla out of bed in the morning to get ready for school (which had been unlike her in the past), so she was concerned her daughter might have a sleeping disorder.

When she walked into my office, Kayla had her head down and was texting on her phone. About six months ago, her dad had purchased a new smartphone for her as a Christmas gift, a reward for her excellent grades. When I asked about Kayla's phone, her mom stated that she had been on her phone a lot more since she had a smartphone.

After examining Kayla, I found that she was a healthy teenager, and she didn't have any other medical conditions. She was very pleasant and showed no tonsil enlargement, which can be the cause of sleep apnea in children. Kayla did not admit to taking any illicit drugs, and her labs were normal. Since I had eliminated virtually every other possible cause for her sleepiness, I turned to look at her sleep habits.

I asked Kayla if she would keep a Sleep Journal and complete a Sleep Assessment, which she agreed to do. When she returned these to me, the data revealed that she was only sleeping an average of six hours and 10 minutes a night.

The culprit? Kayla's unregulated cell phone use.

She was staying up late at night to talk to her friends on social media, and the habit was significantly cutting into her sleep time. Her parents were completely unaware of the fact she was on her phone late at night—sometimes till midnight. Her screen time usage was over five hours a day. As shocking as it may sound, these numbers are not unusual.

According to the American Academy of Child and Adolescent Psychiatry, *children in the US spend between four and six hours a day on screens. Teens can spend up to nine hours.*[151]

Kayla's case is a clear example of how sleep deprivation and insufficient sleep can affect academic performance and family relationships. Cell phone usage—and especially being on social media—has become a huge issue among teens and adolescents.

Unfortunately, parents with the best intentions give their children smartphones and forget to properly regulate how they use them.

In addition, some children can become addicted to their smartphones and manipulate their parents into letting them use the devices without any kind of meaningful supervision. As they spend more time on their devices, the time to perform daily routines—including homework and sleep—gets diminished.

Additionally, spending so much time on their phones can create stress and anxiety from social media usage, not to mention bullying. It can also cause circadian rhythm misalignment, making it harder to fall asleep when they finally do go to bed.

Because most parents attend office visits with their teenagers if they're under the age of 18, it can be hard to get honest answers out of children and teens. If their parents are present, teens tend to give the "right" answer instead of admitting the full extent of their screen time and sleep issues.

In Kayla's case, I recommended restricting her smartphone usage from five hours down to two hours per day. I also requested that she continue maintaining her Sleep Journal so that we could continue to track how much sleep she was getting and adjust her sleep habits as needed.

While it was tough to cut down her screen time at first, with positive reinforcement and support from her family she was able to get her time down to a reasonable amount. Now, Kayla is earning higher grades and feeling better. I continue to see her at my practice so that she will maintain her good sleep habits.

In most cases, I need to enlist the parents' help to get children and teens on track with their sleep habits. And though it's easy for teenagers to revert to their old ways when they head to college, I still strongly encourage them to prioritize sleep between 10 p.m. and 6 a.m., keep a fixed schedule, and follow my *7 Proven Sleep Strategies*.

Delayed Sleep Phase Disorder

Delayed sleep phase disorder (DSPS) is a "clock problem." Children with DSPS have normal sleep duration, quality, and consistency. The problem is simply that their sleep onset is delayed by two or more hours compared to the societal norm. This is because the internal clock (the circadian rhythm) is shifted later during the night.

Per se, DSPS is a rare disorder but it's prevalent among teenagers and is behaviorally induced. They tend to go to bed late and wake up later in the mornings. The incidence of behaviorally induced DSPS is 7–16% among teens and young adults.[152] There is also a familial and genetic component.[153] Folks who are so-called night owls likely suffer from DSPS.

In most cases, DSPS is behaviorally induced due to the habit of going to bed late, especially among teenagers who stay up late. Once teens make a habit of these behaviors, their bodies adapt to this later schedule.[154] When that happens, normal sleep-inducing processes, like the production of melatonin or the dropping of the body core temperature, which promotes sleep, become delayed. This shift in the internal clock is hard to reverse when teens need to wake up early for school.

To make things worse, teenage hormonal changes also shift the clock forward. The combination of their hormonal shifts with their habits makes it tough to sync their body clocks with the outside world's earlier schedule.[155]

The common symptoms are trouble falling asleep and waking up at societal normal times. Also, children or teens with DSPS are tired in the morning and have a tough time waking up at earlier hours. Most children with DSPS also have impaired alertness—especially in the mornings—and suffer from excessive sleepiness and fatigue.[156]

Most of the time, the diagnosis can be established by history taking. Using the enclosed Sleep Journal and Sleep Assessment (which you can also download at SleepFixAcademy.com) will help you document the hours of sleep your child gets and will show the pattern of delayed sleep onset and delayed waking up. It is important to rule out other sleep, medical, mental, or substance abuse disorders. Very rarely, a sleep study is needed to rule out other sleep disorders that can coexist.

The treatment strategy for DSPS involves behavioral therapy, sticking to sleep schedule, as well as resetting the circadian rhythm clock by using **light-box therapy** and melatonin. The light therapy is administered for 30 minutes in the morning upon awakening, and that shifts the clock backward. This therapy requires consistent use and must be administered under the guidance of a sleep specialist. Also, low doses of melatonin at bedtime can help with sleep onset and move the body's clock back.

There is also another treatment called chronotherapy. If moving the clock backward is not feasible, then the strategy is to move it forward to get the rhythm synchronized. Every three to six days, the sleeping time is advanced by two hours till the desired sleep time is achieved. This therapy, too, should only be performed under the guidance of a sleep specialist.

Academic Impact of Insufficient Sleep in Teens

As we saw in Kayla's case, insufficient sleep can wreak havoc on a young person's ability to function. The effects of sleep deprivation—or short sleep, as some researchers call it—extend to virtually all areas of a child's development. It affects mood, learning, behavior, and relationships. One of the most significant effects of short sleep in children seems to be a reduced ability to learn and perform well in school.

According to a 2013 study in the journal *Sleep*, children who reported a shorter sleep duration than the recommended amount showed a shorter attention span and poorer academic performance than their peers who consistently got enough sleep.

The study was conducted in Buenos Aires, Argentina, and used the pediatric daytime sleepiness scale[157] in over 1,000 school children (13–17 years old). Academic performance was measured by gathering literature and math grades. Just as researchers expected, there was a clear association with daytime sleepiness from lack of sleep and poorer academic performance.[158]

Similarly, an Australian study conducted that same year showed that sleep quality and circadian chronotype also played an important role in how teenage students felt and performed during the day. This study found that students with evening chronotypes (night owls) tended to sleep worse and have poorer academic outcomes than their peers. They also reported a more depressed mood.[159]

Even though these studies are over a decade old, they have given us valuable information. And if these studies were to be conducted now, I bet the numbers would be much worse.

Becoming a night owl is increasingly common in teenagers due to the natural hormonal changes in puberty. These changes move the clock forward, creating behaviorally induced delayed sleep phase (going to bed and waking up late), which we discussed previously.[160] This natural phenomenon is compounded by the habit of going to bed late, especially among teenagers who stay up late for many reasons. Eventually, this becomes the norm.

Many teens are misdiagnosed with insomnia because they have difficulty initiating sleep when, in actuality, their internal clock has moved forward. We now know that sleep is induced by the release of melatonin and the core body temperature dropping. In teenagers, poor sleep routines and natural hormonal shifts interfere with this process, and hence, sleep onset is delayed.

For teens suffering from poor sleep quality and insufficient sleep duration, sleep-positive routines should be implemented early on to help mitigate some of the common causes of poor sleep.

If teens go to sleep late (around 11:30 p.m.), they need to sleep at least until 7:30 a.m. to meet the *minimum* sleep requirement for their age and thus prevent insufficient sleep. But to get to school, they usually have to wake up earlier than 7:30. Thus, most teens invariably suffer from insufficient sleep, leading to poor school performance, weight gain, increased depressive symptoms, and motor vehicle accidents.

After looking at available data, the American Academy of Sleep Medicine recommended in 2017 to delay school start time till 8.30 a.m. for middle school and high school students.

In my experience, most teens would be thrilled at the chance for a later school start—and the parents trying to get them out of bed in the morning would be equally happy! It may take the educational system a while to get on board with the idea (it is a complex system after all) but it could make a huge difference in the productivity and quality of life for teens.[161]

Chapter 10

Sleep and Women

Laura was *miserable* all night long and didn't know what to do.

She was only 53 years old so she thought she was too young for menopause, but she just couldn't sleep because she was waking up in the middle of the night *drenched* with sweat.

She tried everything she could think of to help her sleep: she turned the thermostat down to 66 degrees, she drank a special tea at 9 p.m. that was supposed to make her drowsy, and she had even covered up all sources of light in her room.

Laura took multiple supplements that were supposed to help her sleep, including multivitamins, magnesium, valerian root, melatonin, and a chlorophyll liquid. She also tried taking various over-the-counter sleep medications.

But the same thing happened, night after night.

She'd get hot and kick off the covers. But then the perspiration would evaporate, and she would start to freeze. So, she'd pull the covers back over herself and try to go back to sleep.

But as soon as she'd finally dozed off, she'd feel like she needed to urinate, and getting up to go to the bathroom would wake her up even more.

Once again, she'd get into bed, pull the covers up and try to go back to sleep. She'd just begin to doze off, and then it would start all over. . .

For several reasons—including hormonal challenges, such as in Laura's case, or environmental factors like a partner snoring—women have more difficulty sleeping than men.

These sleep differences begin quite early for women, often shortly after adolescence.[162] In fact, research shows that while women are less likely to struggle with sleep apnea, they are at a much higher risk for insomnia compared to their male counterparts.[163] In fact, insomnia is up to two times more common in women than in men. So, why do women bear the brunt of sleep problems? There are quite a few factors at play.

Hormonal Issues

It shouldn't come as much surprise, but hormones play a role in sleep regulation, and hormonal changes can also make sleep elusive. The National Institute of Health estimates that 16–42% of premenopausal women and 39–47% women in menopause experience sleep disturbances.[164]

Even young women report poorer sleep the week before their menstrual cycle,[165] and women with severe premenstrual syndrome (PMS) report more significant sleep disturbances like bad dreams, fatigue, and a lack of concentration due to poor sleep quality.[166]

Most women experience some level of sleep disturbance the week before their period starts.[167] This is caused by hormone-related changes in sleep architecture and usually resolves once menstruation begins. Women may feel more bloated, achy, depressed, and irritable in the days before their period.

The most common treatment for this is over-the-counter pain medicine. Some women report that heating pads, caffeine, eating red meat (due to the body's cravings potentially caused by low iron), and chocolate can help soothe the discomfort—both physically and emotionally—during this time.

Some women have a more severe form of PMS called premenstrual dysphoric disorder, which also tends to cause sleeplessness. On the upside, estrogen and progesterone protect women from sleep apnea; hence, there is less incidence of sleep apnea in premenopausal women.

These issues can also become compounded later in life when women experience hormonal shifts due to perimenopause and menopause.

When women reach menopause, insomnia often gets worse. A study published in July 2018 in the *Journal of Clinical Sleep Medicine* looked at sleep disturbances in women at the cusp of menopause and found the sleep quality was worse for perimenopausal women (or women in menopause) than for those who were premenopausal.[168] Plus hot flashes and night sweats are more common in menopause.

When women enter menopause, their estrogen level decreases, which can put them at risk for more urinary tract infections. Researchers found that the decreased estrogen levels associated with menopausal transition can affect the lining of the urinary passage, thus slowing the movement, resulting in more urinary tract infections. Infections, in turn, result in increased urinary frequency, which causes many nighttime awakenings. These symptoms are worse in women who have a dramatic loss of hormones after surgery to remove ovaries for various reasons, like cancer or cysts.

Most women gain at least five to seven pounds during perimenopause or menopause. If too much weight is gained, women may be at risk for sleep apnea, which, in turn, can make sleep quality worse. Lifestyle changes like getting more exercise and eating a nutrient-dense diet can help mitigate the risk factors for sleep apnea.[169]

Night Sweats

It's not unusual to sweat a bit at night, but soaking your pajamas or sheets is another story. Several issues can cause night sweats, including illness, menopause, or medication side effects. Some common antidepressant medications, like SSRIs, may also cause this symptom as a side effect.[170]

Night sweats can also be related to lifestyle factors, like weight and diet. Drinking excessive alcohol or caffeine can also trigger night sweats.[171] You're also more likely to suffer from night sweats if you sleep in a warm or use heat-retaining bedding.[172]

Maintaining a healthy weight, avoiding excess alcohol, and keeping the thermostat on low may help prevent this frustrating symptom. (It may be surprising, but night sweats are also a symptom of sleep apnea.)

Menopause-related night sweats are caused by hormonal shifts that effect the body's ability to regulate its own temperature. While some medications are approved to treat these night sweats, it's best to try natural solutions first. Try drinking cold water at night and using a cooling mattress or pillow. Getting adequate exercise each day and moderating stress will also lessen the frequency and intensity of night sweats.

If you suspect your night sweats are a symptom of menopause, consult your primary care physician.

Remember Laura's dilemma? When she came to see me, she had been trying several options to try and improve her sleep quality, but nothing helped.

We did a sleep study (results: she didn't have sleep apnea). Lab work indicated she had attained menopause. Hers was a classic example of a perimenopausal woman who is experiencing sleep issues related to her changing hormones, so her physician placed Laura on hormone replacement therapy, which limited her night sweats.

Using the Sleep Journal, Laura started tracking her nightly sleep. Meanwhile, I helped Laura wean herself off the over-the-counter sleep medications she had been taking, and she decided to use her multivitamins twice a week instead of every day. She came to understand that the tea she was drinking could also be a diuretic, causing her to wake up at night to go to the bathroom. So Laura resorted to drinking her favorite tea in the morning instead.

Three months later, when I saw her for a follow-up visit, she was getting good, consolidated sleep for six-and-a-half hours a night. Although not an ideal eight hours, it was better than the disrupted 3–5 hours she was getting when she first came to my office.

Mood Disorders

Mood disorders like anxiety and depression are more prevalent in women and lead to more sleep disruptions. In fact, women are twice as likely as men to experience major depression at some point in their lives. Researchers believe that this difference is due to both hormonal and societal factors.

In addition to having to ride out their monthly hormonal ebbs and flows and then endure menopause, women also shoulder more family burdens than men. They're more likely to take care of domestic duties, including childrearing, cooking, cleaning, and caring for parents as they age.

Young teen girls and women are also more vulnerable to the effects of social media and the perils of bullying. According to a recent report from *Common Sense Media*, teens spend an average of seven hours and 22 minutes using screens each day.[173] This can result in anxiety and can cause significant issues with sleep.

In addition to simply throwing off their circadian rhythm, increased scrolling is linked to a more depressed mood in adolescent girls. Excessive social media usage is also correlated with a more negative body image and an increased risk of suicidal thoughts.

For patients whose mood disorders are affecting their sleep, I recommend seeing a mental health specialist who may recommend treatments like talk therapy, mindfulness exercises, or medication. In cases of mental illness, treating the underlying condition before adding sleep aids is always the best approach.

Pregnancy

Most women experience fragmented sleep as pregnancy progresses and once they're caring for their newborn. Sleep is challenging in pregnancy for several reasons.

Pregnancy can be associated with a constant urge to move the legs due to RLS. Although it may seem counterintuitive, the symptoms of RLS are worsened by rest and gets better with movement. Up to 30% of pregnant women suffer from this condition, and it is more common in the third trimester due to the depletion of iron from the growing fetus.

As I mentioned previously, iron deficiency is the most common cause of RLS, and symptoms can be treated with iron supplementation. If iron therapy is not helping, there are FDA-approved foot vibrating devices for the treatment of RLS. Other commonly used medications to treat RLS are contraindicated in pregnancy. Thankfully, RLS associated with pregnancy usually resolves once the baby is born.

Snoring is also more likely when a woman is pregnant due to weight gain and hormonal changes. If there are symptoms of snoring during pregnancy, it is important to rule out sleep apnea as it can be detrimental both to mom and the unborn fetus due to the lack of oxygen during apneic episodes.

Aside from these issues, general discomfort also interferes with sleep during pregnancy. Women may not be able to sleep in their favorite positions due to their growing baby bump, and quality of sleep is affected due to back pain or leg cramps.

Pregnant women also may need to wake up to urinate more frequently because of pressure on their bladder from their expanding uterus. In addition, pregnant women may experience more stress and worry due to the anticipation of labor and newborn caregiving.

As challenging as it is to obtain, sleep is crucial for pregnant women. Women who got six or fewer hours of sleep during pregnancy showed increased inflammatory markers and had a higher risk of preeclampsia, gestational diabetes, and unplanned Cesarean deliveries.[174]

While there are not many quick fixes for pregnant women, and most medications are off-limits, there are still options for pregnant women.

Short naps are recommended during pregnancy to combat poor sleep at night. A study in the *Journal of Clinical Sleep Medicine* reported that shorter naps (shorter than 90 minutes) are more beneficial for overall sleep quality at night than longer naps.[175] Naps over 90 minutes were associated with impaired nighttime sleep quality and continuity.

One study also found that women who began practicing **mindfulness meditation** and *hatha* yoga classes during their second trimester enjoyed better sleep throughout the rest of their pregnancy.[176]

These interventions are best started early in pregnancy when most problems arise. The same study noted that women who started these same exercises in their third trimester did not see an improvement in sleep.

And as most moms experience after the birth of their child, sleep unfortunately does not immediately improve. New mothers report a significant drop in sleep satisfaction after they give birth, due to the newborn's frequent awakenings.[177] Women who breastfeed report even lower sleep satisfaction since they get up multiple times in the night to feed their baby.[178]

Some mothers don't reach their pre-child sleep satisfaction levels until six years after giving birth.[179] For this reason, I recommend using the *7 Proven Sleep Strategies* to improve and recoup as much lost sleep as possible during this time.

The Vigilance of Caregiving

Tara was a 32-year-old mom with a three-year-old son, Caden, and a 16-month-old daughter, Ellie Rose. Tara was active in her community of moms with preschoolers, ate a balanced diet, and exercised regularly—she had even trained for and run her first half marathon. Still, she was exhausted.

Tara's husband traveled for work, so she was a single parent three to four nights a week. On those nights, it took her a good hour and a half to bathe Caden and Ellie, read to them, and rock her baby girl to sleep. Then she'd clean the kitchen and collapse on the couch with a glass of wine to watch a TV show or two. She was exhausted but couldn't turn off her mind. Most nights it was close to midnight before Tara went to sleep.

But Ellie was an early riser. At 5:30 a.m. on the dot, her cries would reverberate through the baby monitor. Tara would *will* her body out of bed, shuffle to the baby's room, get her daughter from her crib, and head back to the main bedroom, stopping by the kitchen on the way to grab a banana for the baby.

Back in her bedroom, Tara would secure a spot in the middle of the bed for Ellie to eat the banana. And if Tara was lucky, she herself would doze just a few more minutes while Ellie played.

On Saturdays, when Tara's husband was home, he'd take the morning shift so Tara could sleep a little longer. But week after week, averaging just five and a half hours of sleep per night, her sleep debt was adding up quickly.

Tara became more anxious and nervous, even short-tempered. She met with a counselor to address the anxiety, but she knew what she needed most was more sleep.

She often wondered how she could get her mind to wind down faster so she could get to sleep sooner, and how she could get back to sleep after attending to a scared or sick kid in the middle of the night.

☾

Tara's not alone. Research has clearly shown sleep problems are more prevalent in women, and my personal and clinical experience confirms this as well. Because women are natural nurturers and protectors, they maintain a heightened state of alertness all the time. This is especially true at night.

Women are often the "default parent," meaning they tend to be the one who hears the baby cry for feeding, be aware of the teenager sneaking out, or even be the one who wakes up because of the neighbor's dog barking late at night.

There were many mornings my wife told me that the children came home past their curfew or that there was an overnight thunderstorm. I was often oblivious, possibly because I was recovering from an on-call night during my ICU days, and such disturbances were simply not on my radar.

Likewise, when I was a teenager, my mother often expressed that she had many sleepless nights, likely in part because she was worried about my brother, sister, and me.

Women seem to have a strong caregiving instinct—a gift that can also be a curse when it comes to getting good rest. In an ideal world, I'd encourage Tara to enlist more help from her spouse and family. But that may not always be available. Whether your spouse travels for work, is someone who works shifts, or you're a single parent, often the responsibilities fall to one person.

Where should you start? First, let's talk about winding down for sleep. Like Tara, you may find yourself tired but wired. If Tara would have come to me when her kids were little, I would have talked to her about my *7 Proven Sleep Strategies*.

Not only would they have helped her establish a good sleep plan and calm her mind; they would also help her go back to sleep faster when one of the kids woke up at night. So often, caregivers are woken up in the middle of the night. A child wakes from a bad dream or suddenly sick. A mom may be up for just a few minutes or an hour, and now the challenge is getting back to sleep.

If that's the case for you, the meditation, mindfulness, and Vivid Imagination® exercises I offer later in the book can help you sleep better. Of course, you can also enlist the help of your spouse and family to share this burden more equally.

Sometimes the biggest issue is your children's sleep habits. Addressing issues like we discussed in Chapter 8 (Sleep and Children) might help you find the root cause of extra caregiving. Whether it's addressing childhood sleep apnea, or enforcing curfew with your teen, either way getting help for your kids can help you both get the sleep you need. Sometimes, that includes taking a nap. We'll discuss sleep debt and naps in Chapter 12 (Sleep, Performance, and Success).

Environmental Sleep Disorder

Women are also more likely to suffer from environmental sleep disorder. This occurs when you can't sleep because of an external problem—like your partner snoring, loud noises outside, or even the temperature in the room being too high or too low. Environmental sleep disorder is especially common in minorities who are more likely to live in areas with higher traffic, artificial light, and noise.[180]

This hyperawareness is likely linked to women's role as caregivers, as mentioned before. Their bodies are wired to wake them up due to even small noises or disturbances as it could be a sign that their family is in danger, even once their children are grown.

It's very common in my practice to meet couples who are sleeping apart (a sleep divorce) because of snoring. The good news is that environmental factors are often easier to manipulate than internal ones. If you struggle with environmental sleep disorder, consider assessing your bedroom and creating a sleep haven.

If your partner is in denial that he snores, one popular way to help him comprehend the problem is to use your smartphone to record the nighttime snoring. Armed with undeniable audio evidence, many women are able to give their spouse perspective when he actually hears how loud his snoring is.

Environmental sleep disorder typically resolves once the disturbance is removed. Another way to decrease your risk for environmental sleep disorder is to increase your exposure to nature and experience more natural light during the day.

Just because women are more predisposed to sleep issues doesn't mean they should just accept their sleep-deprived state. Whatever is hindering sleep in your life—whether it's hormone-related shifts, environmental disruptions, stress, or parenting—help is available.

Treating insomnia begins with reworking your sleep habits and treating all underlying conditions that may contribute to sleep problems. If you're doing everything right and are *still* struggling to get a good night's sleep, schedule a consultation with a sleep doctor today.

Chapter 11

Sleep and Older Adults

Carlos was a 74-year-old gentleman with a long history of sleep apnea. He had been using his CPAP consistently for several years and was doing well before he came to see me.

Since he hadn't been sleeping well, his daughter Emilia, whom I'd known for many years, brought him in for a checkup.

Unfortunately, Carlos's wife of 52 years, Maria, had recently passed away after a prolonged illness. He admitted to being lonely after her passing. Carlos and Maria used to play cards together and enjoy evening walks hand in hand.

In the six months since her passing, Carlos didn't have a routine anymore. He frequently took naps during the day and spent most of the time indoors. He also admitted he had crying spells when he thought of Maria, and that he'd completely stopped going to church, which had been his significant social lifeline.

Carlos seemed rather withdrawn and, according to Emilia, he was not his usual self. On the positive side, Carlos was still using his CPAP machine regularly.

During an evaluation, it became evident that most of his symptoms were rooted in his loss of companionship resulting in a lack of routine. His new habit of drinking more beer than usual at night while watching TV wasn't helping either.

I encouraged Carlos to keep a Sleep Journal and complete a Sleep Assessment to document his sleep and report back to me. Medically, everything looked good, but I could tell he needed some intervention to help him adjust to his new life without his beloved wife.

I took the liberty of "prescribing" that he find someone he could talk with and recommended that he enroll in the local senior center. He agreed.

Emilia was able to arrange a consultation with a counselor to address his symptoms of sadness and loneliness (very common in older folks, especially after they lose their loved ones). I also advised him to walk regularly in the evenings.

He was able to do all this, and at his follow-up appointment a few months later, Carlos seemed to be in a much better place. Emilia was relieved that her dad was doing better emotionally and was encouraged that he had also joined the pickle ball team at the senior center.

By addressing specific issues and making minor adjustments to his routine, Carlos was able to adapt even to this major loss. Fortunately, he also had a loving family, including his daughter Emilia, who was intimately involved in his care.

☽

When in a frantically busy stage of life, many people look forward to retirement as a time when they can finally get some sleep.

Unfortunately, by the age that most people have fewer claims on their time, they've lost their natural ability to sleep through the night. Overall, sleep quality worsens with every decade of life, and by the time you reach 70, total sleep time and quality of sleep is often not optimal.

And as you age, life changes can throw your routine off and create sleep problems.

While adults aged 70 and older need roughly the same amount of sleep as younger adults—seven to eight hours—many struggle to get sufficient sleep. When they are able to doze off, they spend more time in lighter stages of sleep. There are many reasons (some of which are discussed below) for this sleep slump, including medical and behavioral issues that can compound sleep difficulties.

Advanced Sleep Phase Disorder

With aging comes biological changes in the brain that can alter your sleep pattern. Older adults sometimes go to bed as early as 6–8 p.m. and then wake up as early as 2–3 a.m. This is called ASPS, the result of an alteration in the SCN, which, as you may recall, regulates the circadian rhythm. Simply put, if you go to bed too early, you wake up too early.

The incidence of ASPS is rare, about 1% in middle-aged and older adults.[181] The exact cause is unknown, but in older people, it is usually behaviorally induced.

According to *Stanford Medicine*, genetics can play a role. About 40–50% of people who suffer from ASPS have a relative with the same condition.[182] Though there's certainly a biological component to ASPS, behavioral factors are believed to be the main contributors to this problem.

Retirees and those who don't have responsibilities that keep them occupied are especially vulnerable to ASPS. Loneliness also plays a role in their mental state.

Coincidentally, in May 2023, Surgeon General Dr. Vivek Murthy labeled loneliness and isolation as an under-appreciated public health crisis, stating that "loneliness and isolation increase the risk for individuals to develop mental health challenges in their lives, and lacking connection can increase the risk for premature death to levels comparable to smoking daily."[183] For retirees, the connection with ASPS is evident.

Without a packed schedule, older folks tend to take daytime naps, which in turn affects the ability to have consolidated sleep at night.

After a few months, the habit of going to bed early, waking up early, and taking long naps becomes the routine. Their early-bird schedule quickly becomes a major inconvenience, as they wake up early and then have significant daytime sleepiness.

Extremely early wake-up times can also exacerbate mental health struggles like depression. It can also disrupt other family members who are trying to sleep.

If left untreated, ASPS can cause long-term sleep deprivation. Folks with ASPS may push themselves to go to bed later, but without treatment and changes in sleep habits, they will continue to wake up quite early. When this compounds over time, people can rack up a large sleep debt.

The **treatment for ASPS** involves first understanding the sleep pattern. In my clinic, I offer clients a Sleep Journal and Sleep Assessment so we can track when sleep onset most frequently occurs when a person goes to bed, each nighttime awakening, when they wake up in the morning, or if there are other reasons affecting their sleep quality. Once we have this information in hand, it's easier to see where they have gotten off track.

Once we have identified a target bedtime and wake time, we begin shifting the clock forward by using **light-box therapy** closer to bedtime at night, usually for about 30 minutes around 7 p.m. This tricks the SCN into thinking it is still daytime. Eventually, this method pushes the internal clock forward to the desired sleep time. *Such treatment should only be administered by a practitioner with expertise in sleep medicine.*

Finally, medications like **melatonin** can be helpful if given closer to bedtime to initiate sleep earlier and to increase sleep time. Once a person has their sleep time back on track, I advise they **keep a strict sleep schedule** (usually from 10 p.m. to 6 a.m.) every night. It also helps to avoid bright sunlight till after 10 a.m. to prevent phase shifting backward, cut out all caffeine after their morning cup of coffee, and avoid taking afternoon naps.

This maintenance ensures the clock shift is permanent; otherwise, people can easily revert back to the advanced sleep schedule.

Sleep and Medical and Psychological Problems

Multiple medical problems can alter sleep, and since older adults tend to have more medical issues, sleep can become a challenge. Part of my treatment of older adults involves working with their primary care doctor to resolve their other health problems so that sleep can flourish.

Medical problems that interfere with sleep run the gamut. Poorly controlled diabetes and prostate or bladder issues can result in frequent urination that makes people wake up multiple times a night.

Cardiovascular problems can cause shortness of breath, especially when lying flat, which can also cause multiple awakenings. Breathing problems like asthma and COPD sometimes compromise sleep for a number of reasons, including frequent coughing, difficulty breathing, and wheezing. Other medical conditions, like acid reflux and dementia, can result in poor quality of sleep.

It's not just physical issues that erode sleep quality. Mental health in older individuals also plays a role in how well—or how poorly—they sleep at night.

Anxiety and depression can cause awakenings, resulting in poor sleep quality and insomnia. Insomnia, in turn, can worsen anxiety. As in Carlos's case, older people may experience loneliness or isolation, and this can cause or worsen symptoms of insomnia.

They also tend to spend more time indoors, especially if they live in assisted living or long-term care or skilled nursing facilities without much light exposure. These environments can worsen internal-clock-related sleep problems.

Some folks resort to drinking alcohol to induce sleep, and some may even try substances like marijuana for quick relief of their insomnia. Unfortunately, these are not long-term solutions and can worsen insomnia over time. What's more, these habits can lead to dependence or even substance abuse.

To complicate matters even further, some medications that older adults take to manage other health conditions can also interfere with sleep. Diuretics cause people to use the restroom more frequently at night, and medications to treat hypertension, like beta blockers, can affect sleep quality and duration. (It can help taking diuretics and beta blockers in the morning, if possible.)

Chronic pain—from low back, neck, shoulder, and other areas—can also significantly alter sleep. These aches need to be addressed with a primary care doctor or physical therapist.

Though they face more challenges than my younger clients, my older clients typically have more available time and resources to work on their sleep. By addressing the various medical and mental conditions they experience, adults 70 years and older can markedly improve their sleep.

Also, by addressing their sleep conditions, older individuals can mitigate the risk of mental decline. Sleep apnea is one of the risk factors for dementia and is also prevalent in this age group.[184] Sleep apnea is treatable, though. That's why I recommend that people with suspected sleep apnea seek out a sleep study sooner rather than later.

Treatment for Insomnia in Older Adults

My *7 Proven Sleep Strategies* can help improve anyone's sleep, and they tend to be effective in older adults. However, folks over 70 years old may need additional treatment to resolve their sleep issues.

One of the most effective treatment methods is CBT for insomnia (CBT-I). CBT-I helps folks change their negative associations with sleep or the bedroom, so that they reduce their sleep anxiety from previous bouts of insomnia. It also helps them restrict their sleep schedule, so that they're not spending too many hours in bed, which can also contribute to insomnia.

A recent study found that engaging in CBT-I—or the truncated version of the same therapy, known as brief behavioral therapy for insomnia—significantly improved sleep quality for many participants.[185] If a person has tried improving their sleep hygiene and is still unable to sleep, it may be worth seeing a specialist who can administer one of these therapies.

That said, with some intentionality and diligence, adults over 70 can get their sleep back on track. Older adults should implement healthy habits, like regular exercise, a healthy diet, limited screen time, and regular waking and bedtimes to optimize their sleep.

Like anyone, if sleep issues persist, it may be worth consulting with a sleep specialist to see if there's another underlying issue at play.

Chapter 12

Sleep, Performance, and Success

Sleep and Work

Theresa came into my office and burst into tears. Her life was falling apart, and she was about to get fired. She had always been told she was a great employee, but now she just couldn't seem to focus, and the pressure at work had been creeping up on her. She was scared and in a panic.

She was in her early 50s and was a high-performing executive with a highly stressful job. To her credit, Theresa had beaten a dependence on prescription drugs early in her career and had fully recovered. In the past, she had used zolpidem for insomnia, ativan (typically used for anxiety, but she used it to sleep), and even trazadone to help her sleep. They had all ultimately failed, and she wanted to avoid any temptation to revert to her previous medication dependence.

Although she admitted she was "drinking a little too much wine" to help her fall asleep at night, she was clear about not wanting to be prescribed any more medications to fall asleep. I fully supported her concern.

Working together, we were able to pinpoint exactly when her symptoms started, which was shortly after her divorce. This dramatic **precipitating event** caused her to lose sleep. Such events include any events that we typically have no control over—job loss, divorce, or the death of a loved one, for example. These commonly trigger short-term sleep loss; however, the symptoms should resolve after the impact of the event has faded.

Theresa's sleep loss was compounded by **perpetuating habits**, especially having several glasses of wine before bed, watching TV shortly before bed, and keeping her iPad right on her bedside table. She also had some sleep-positive and neutral routines: having background noise cancellation technology and doing meditation prior to bedtime. (Perpetuating habits also include worrying about sleep and consistently using alcohol or sleeping pills. Once such bad habits are in place, insomnia is harder to resolve.)

And as a woman in mid-life, Theresa could naturally be **predisposed** to sleep disruptions because of menopause-related hormonal factors, but in her case, hormonal changes did not play a role.

After asking her to keep a Sleep Journal and complete a Sleep Assessment, we were able to identify the root causes of her insomnia and work to resolve them. This involved speaking with a therapist about her divorce and some lingering anxiety from her childhood and breaking the sleep-negative routine of self-medicating with alcohol.

Once she made these changes, her sleep improved drastically—and soon, her overall health did too. After six months, Theresa lost 30 pounds, had more energy than ever, and was even given a promotion at work.

In today's environment, work stress is one of the leading causes for poor quality of sleep. The working-from-home trend, in particular, has resulted in a lack of boundaries between work and rest. Many folks even work on their laptops in bed, making it difficult to fall asleep at night.

Men, women, and professionals who hold high-authority positions are especially susceptible to the constant pressure to perform and make tough decisions. The stress they are under is tremendous, and this, in turn, results in them working longer, which cuts into the total sleep time. And for some, much of their free time is spent worrying about the tough decisions they must make.

Sleep and Productivity: Disasters in the Night

On the night of April 14, 1912, the crew of the *Titanic* spotted a massive iceberg. It was peeking through the still, freezing waters of the North Atlantic, and the ship and its thousands of passengers were floating right toward it.

"Iceberg, dead ahead!" yelled lookout Frederick Fleet.

First Officer William Murdoch looked where Fleet was pointing and quickly noticed the huge iceberg. Murdoch, who was captaining the ship, had only a split second to decide how to avoid the obstacle. After a second's hesitation, he gave the order to reverse the engine and turn the ship sharply to the right.[186]

This proved to be a *disastrous* choice.

The steam engine couldn't reverse this quickly, and so the engine was effectively halted. With its reduced speed, the ship couldn't turn sharply or quickly enough, and it continued to drift toward the iceberg.

It's widely believed that had Murdoch turned while maintaining the ship's previous speed instead of slowing it, the *Titanic* would have narrowly avoided the collision—and the disaster of epic proportions.[187]

The time of the collision was 11:40 p.m.

Historians have speculated for over a century about this fateful decision. Did the crew need more training? A better lookout system?

There's no proven fact that sleep deprivation was involved, but as a sleep doctor, my first thought is whether such a miscalculation was, in fact, related to sleep deprivation since it occurred so late at night.

Of course, we'll never know the answer with any degree of certainty. However, I do know there's an abundance of evidence suggesting that our reflexes and response rates are drastically diminished at night.

Mishaps involving naval aircraft destroyers *Fitzgerald* and *John S. McCain* were attributed in part to sleep-deprived crew members.[188] A study by the National Highway Safety Administration reveals that almost 50% of fatal car accidents happen at night, even though only about 25% of motor vehicles are on the road during the night hours.[189]

This is because drivers who are on the road late at night are more likely to experience the effects of fatigue, including excessive sleepiness, lower alertness, slower reaction time, alcohol consumption, and a tendency to fall asleep at the wheel.[190] In fact, "almost 20% of all serious car crash injuries in the general population are associated with driver sleepiness, independent of alcohol effects."[191]

Lack of sleep can be a ticking time bomb.

Insomnia results in tremendous economic loss.

Workers with insomnia are more likely to report irritability, poor concentration, diminished short-term memory, and a lack of energy to accomplish their tasks. Chronic sleep deprivation is also associated with negative work outcomes, including occupational errors, accidents and absenteeism.[192]

Compared to people who don't have sleep issues, "insomniacs reported more medical problems, had more physician-office visits, were hospitalized twice as often, and used more medication."[193] According to the 2012 American Insomnia Survey, workplace accidents caused by insomnia were much more costly than non-insomnia-related errors. The average cost of insomnia-related accidents was $32,062 per incident, while the average cost of other workplace errors was $21,914.[194]

In addition to these problems, employees with insomnia are more likely not to show up at work at all, an average loss of 45–54 days in workplace productivity per year.[195] According to a study reported as early as in 2006, the absenteeism rate for insomniacs was 1.4 times higher than their counterparts.[196]

If a worker is absent from work, not only will that individual forfeit income (assuming they don't have paid time off), but the company will also lose labor, thus affecting them financially. The economic impact of insomnia or other sleep disorders in 2021 was estimated to be as high as $411 billion.[197, 198]

But even when sleep-deprived workers are present at the office, they are more likely to be anxious, irritable, and less productive. [199] For this reason, as of 2014, the CDC has declared sleep deprivation a public health problem.[200] More than a third of American adults are not getting enough sleep on a regular basis.[201]

In addition to these indirect economic costs, the direct costs of insomnia—outpatient care, sleep studies, over-the-counter medications, and more—are also significant. A 2009 study conducted in Quebec found that the average annual cost of sleeplessness for folks with insomnia syndrome was $5,010 per worker per year.[202]

One number that's difficult to calculate is the *indirect* cost of people self-medicating for their insomnia. Unfortunately, many sleep-deprived people still don't seek healthcare for their insomnia and instead turn to quick-fix remedies like over-the-counter medications, alcohol, or marijuana to induce sleep. These maladaptive behaviors, in turn, create more issues in the long run and often have a negative impact at work.

During the pandemic, the prolific use of electronic gadgets and home-monitoring devices gave out tons of data about sleep quality. The problem lies in how to analyze the data and what can be done about the findings. People tend to worry when their gadget reveals that "they did not get deep sleep last night" and end with sleep anxiety, only making the situation worse. They do online research and often end with *worse* sleep habits, resulting in a lack of quality sleep and more self-medicating.

But poor sleep does not only cost you financially; it can be *fatal.*

Sleep deprivation leads to cognitive impairment and compromises your memory and reflexes. This can lead to more errors and accidents.

A study of nurses revealed that cognitive performance was significantly impaired in night shift workers, and nurses who worked the night shift had a 32% higher chance of mathematical errors than nurses who worked the day shift.[203]

Similarly, truckers with insomnia were shown to have a significantly higher incidence of motor vehicle accidents as compared to their peers who did not suffer from insomnia.[204] In jobs like these, mistakes can result in fatal outcomes with significant financial consequences.[205]

Several major disasters—like the *Titanic*, Three Mile Island (a nuclear reactor at the Three Mile Island nuclear facility in Pennsylvania had a partial meltdown), and the Chernobyl disaster (where one of the nuclear reactors at the Chernobyl nuclear power plant in Ukraine exploded)—all occurred at night.

Terrance

One night, after a 12-hour night shift, Terrance was driving home and veered off the road, causing his SUV to roll over. Thankfully, Terrance escaped unscathed, but his vehicle was totaled. Terrance was an ICU nurse and a former coworker of mine.

When he came to see me and I asked him about the wreck, he admitted he had fallen asleep at the wheel. When he awoke, there was a pedestrian right in front of him, and he overcorrected to avoid the person. While deeply concerned, I wasn't surprised by his accident since *drowsy driving can often be more dangerous than drunk driving.*

Later that week, Terrance came to my office for a consultation, and I diagnosed him with SWSD (shift worker sleep disorder) and started him on an FDA-approved medication for this condition. Thankfully, the medication helped Terrance to adapt to his challenging schedule.

Every year in the US, 1.23 *million* days are lost due to insufficient sleep.[206] The financial impact is enormous, well into the billions of dollars.

If you suffer from sleep deprivation, the good news is that there is help available. In the following chapters, we'll discuss how to form strong sleep strategies that will have you falling asleep faster, staying asleep longer, and waking up feeling rejuvenated. In turn, you'll be able to avoid these perils and perform your best at work.

Pete

Pete was a 57-year-old commercial truck driver who did 18-wheeler long-haul trips up and down the East Coast. Pete's annual medical examination—required by the Department of Transportation (DOT)—showed that he was overweight, had high blood pressure, and he had a neck circumference of 18 inches.[207] (A normal neck circumference of over 17 inches for men is and over 16 inches for women is considered a risk factor for OSA.)

Though these factors might seem unrelated to Pete's driving performance at first glance, a high BMI and a large neck circumference are both correlated with sleep apnea. The frequent disruptions in sleep that happen with sleep apnea can cause daytime drowsiness, which is extremely dangerous for someone in this line of work—*and* for the vehicles around him.

Because of his risk factors, Pete was told he needed a sleep specialist evaluation to rule out sleep apnea and make sure he was safe to drive.

When he came to the office, we asked Pete to complete a sleep-related questionnaire, called the **Epworth sleepiness scale**. The scale asks participants to assign a numerical score representing their drowsiness in several situations, with zero meaning "no chance of falling asleep" and three meaning "having a high chance of falling asleep."

The questionnaire includes everyday circumstances like sitting and reading, watching TV, waiting at a stoplight, as a passenger in an automobile, or sitting quietly after a meal. Once the participant has assigned a numerical answer for each situation, we tally up the score. Scores over 10 are considered significant for sleepiness.

The problem is that the sleep questionnaire is subjective. Commercial drivers who are forced to have evaluations tend to underrate their sleepiness because they don't want to lose their jobs. Pete's score was three, while the national average for truck drivers hovers between three and five for the test.

Despite the low score in the screening tool, I harbored some concerns. Given Pete's high BMI, neck circumference, and hypertension, I suggested we perform further tests. Sure enough, a sleep study confirmed that Pete suffered from sleep apnea.

Truckers are often some of the most reluctant patients, given that they are forced to get tested rather than coming in of their own volition. Plus, their livelihood is at stake.

Under the threat of losing their job, it's sometimes easy to lose sight of what's most important—their health and the safety of those around them on the road.

Though Pete wasn't thrilled at his new diagnosis at first, the DOT has strict criteria. The drivers must be compliant with their therapy to continue to renew their commercial driver's license. Despite his grumbling, Pete's CPAP treatment for sleep apnea made a world of difference.

In the three years since, Pete has been able to keep his job, taper off two of his blood pressure medications, and he even lost 35 pounds. He now wakes up with more energy, feels refreshed, and no longer worries about falling asleep at the wheel.

I recommend that *all* public safety professionals—commercial drivers, pilots, and train engineers—should be screened for sleep disorders if they have risk factors like obesity, high blood pressure, and an increased neck circumference. I believe that this kind of widespread testing will protect public safety.

Most professionals suffering from sleep disorders will feel much happier and more energetic when they address their problem and get the rest they need. Though they sometimes arrive grumbling, with time my patients are happy as they are able to sleep well again—often for the first time in many years.

The Relationship Between Poor Sleep and Accidents at Work

Unfortunately, truck drivers aren't the only workers whose sleep issues create problems. According to the National Sleep Foundation, overwhelming evidence demonstrates that sleep deprivation causes an increase in workplace accidents *across all fields*.

Not surprisingly, sleep-deprived employees are far more likely to have accidents at the workplace than their well-rested counterparts, no matter what type of job they have. Sleep deprivation leads to cognitive impairment,[208] and this, in turn, affects reflexes and reaction times. It also affects judgment and can create a false sense of security, leading to poor decision-making and poorer outcomes. For employees working with the public—train and bus drivers, nurses, and the like—these risks can prove hazardous and tragic.

There are many reasons that so many workers aren't getting enough sleep.

Long hours make it difficult to carve out the time that they need for sleep, and shift workers, in particular, struggle to get adequate rest since they are working against their body's natural rhythm.

In the healthcare industry, there's no way to completely avoid reversed sleep schedules, since hospitals stay open 24/7. Workers at many other industries that have operations 24/7—like first responders, manufacturing, packaging, trucking etc.—are all vulnerable.

Shift work is extremely rough on circadian rhythms. Typically, hospital shifts are 12 hours long, and if you account for signing out, handing over, and travel time, it can be a solid 14–15 hours before a healthcare worker reaches their home.

Imagine working a 7–7 (7 p.m. to 7 a.m.) shift. By the time you get home, it may be nine in the morning. You still need to shower and eat, wind down, and get ready for bed. Even if you are in bed by 10 a.m. and sleep for six hours (provided there are not many interruptions, which are far more common during the day), by the time you wake up, it's 4 p.m. By this point, it's time to start thinking about your next shift.

To make matters worse, most night shift schedules at the hospital alternate between three or four nightshifts in a row, followed by three nights for recovery. As difficult as it is to adjust to a nocturnal schedule in the first place, switching back and forth from week to week is even harder on your body.

Because of this, shift workers are more likely to be chronically sleep-deprived. Their reaction time is simply not as quick compared to folks who work a regular nine-to-five job and get plenty of sleep.[209]

Medical residents in training who, in the past, were assigned on-call shifts, are particularly vulnerable. Fortunately, the Accreditation Council for Graduate Medical Education has taken drastic measures over the past two decades to limit the number of hours the residents can work, although their shifts are still significant and often occur at night.

☽

It's very clear that being sleep-deprived *no matter what you do* can have a tremendous impact on your work performance. You are susceptible to errors and the economic impact of these can be astronomical and even tragic.

And although there are many safety guidelines and screening tools available, it is up to you to make sure you are not sleep-deprived so you can be at your optimum best at work.

Sleep and Athletic Performance

Victor was a 22-year-old lineman who played college football. When traveling with his team, his teammates often heard him screaming in panic in the middle of the night. They also couldn't miss his loud snoring.

His coach had gotten an earful from Victor's teammates—no one wanted to share a room with him during trips away. So, the coach insisted that Victor come to see me for an evaluation.

Victor's mom had also been bugging her son to see a doctor about his sleep issues as she had heard that famous football player Reggie White had died from causes related to sleep apnea. Turns out she had every right to be concerned.

Her son had a big frame. He weighed 234 pounds, and his neck circumference was 19 inches. Even in a younger athlete like Victor, during sleep, the excess fat and tissue around the neck would fall backward due to gravity and constrict the airway. Victor admitted that his girlfriend often told him that he'd stop breathing in his sleep.

His medical history showed significant PTSD and anxiety. I also suspected sleep apnea and I performed a home sleep study, which showed severe sleep apnea.

I also asked Victor to keep a Sleep Journal and Sleep Assessment. These showed that his athletic schedule wasn't helping. Victor exercised late in the evening many nights, but this causes an increase in the secretion of endorphins, which compounded his sleep problems.

His Sleep Journal and Sleep Assessment also showed that, on average, he went to bed at around midnight. It took him a *long* time to fall asleep, and though he woke up at 6:30 or 7 a.m. most days, due to his sleep latency, he was getting less sleep than it seemed at first glance.

When Victor was on the road, his sleep was even worse, with an average of 5.5 hours per night.

I placed him in an insomnia treatment program and addressed his severe sleep apnea. While his weight was a benefit to his college football career, we were able to work on other factors to help make a difference.

The insomnia program included the *7 Proven Sleep Strategies*. For several weeks, he kept a detailed journal of when he slept, woke, drank coffee, exercised, etc. Once I had this information, we worked together to create a routine that would serve him better.

This treatment was based entirely on behavior modification, with no medication required. By addressing his sleep apnea, changing his workout schedule, and improving sleep habits, he was able to perform at his best throughout the season.

When I saw Victor again, he was doing well, and he was performing much better for his team. He was also able to pass this information along to some of his teammates.

Athletes require quality sleep for peak performance, but they're often poor sleepers due to their lifestyles and from the toll of their busy training schedule, frequent travel, musculoskeletal pain, and an increase in core body temperatures from working out. Plus, studies show that athletes have very poor sleep hygiene compared to the general population.[210]

On top of this, college athletes also face academic pressure in addition to their athletic commitments, creating a perfect scenario for poor quality of sleep and sleep deprivation.

Effects of Sleep Deprivation on Athletes

As we know, sleep loss affects virtually every system in the body. For that reason, it's no wonder that athletic performance suffers when players don't get enough sleep or don't get good quality sleep.

Interestingly, a 2015 study noted that lack of sleep in athletes specifically results in several issues:

- It creates an imbalance of the autonomous nervous system, making it difficult for athletes to reach their peak performance.
- Sleep deprivation also may compromise the immune system, putting athletes at a higher risk for getting sick.
- Inadequate sleep resulted in mild cognitive impairment; athletes who were sleep-deprived showed "slower and less accurate" cognitive performance.[211]

In other words, although physical performance remained similar for athletes who were sleep-deprived versus those who weren't, the sleep-deprived participants reacted slower and made worse choices than their peers. And anyone who's played sports—whether at the club level or professionally—knows that the ability to make quick and strategic decisions is key.

Another study found that sleep-deprived athletes had a higher rate of perceived exhaustion compared to their well-rested peers. [212] While it's unclear what effect this subjective measure of fatigue is, the researchers believe that *feeling* tired makes players perform worse than if they feel well rested.

The study found another objective difference between these athletes. The ones who didn't get enough sleep had metabolic disruptions: their bodies showed "altered glucose metabolism and neuroendocrine function [which can] influence an athlete's nutritional, metabolic, and endocrine status negatively and hence potentially reduce athletic performance."[213]

While it sounds minor, this change affects how the muscles are fed, so to speak, which becomes extremely important during strenuous athletic performance. Researchers believe this metabolic change may be due to a lack of human growth hormone (HGH). Normally, HGH is secreted in sleep, but athletes who don't get enough sleep are believed to be deficient in it. HGH also plays an important part in how muscles repair and rebuild themselves, so it makes sense that athletes with compromised sleep would have a decline in performance.

The Third Quarter Slump

I am an avid football fan. I love watching football on TV and, even more, I love sitting in the stands and watching a game live.

Interestingly, my favorite National Football League (NFL) team often plays their games at noon. I often notice a slight lack of effort in the third quarter, which occurs around 1:40 p.m., especially if it is a home game. This is when the other team seems to rack up points against us.

There is also a general lull in the crowd at the same time. I notice this whether I am seeing it on TV or feeling it in arena as a fan. The once-enthusiastic crowd starts to lose steam. The stands begin to be still, and the volume drops inside the stadium.

So, why the sudden drop in energy?

I suspect that the body's circadian rhythm is to blame. Most of us know intuitively that everyone's sleepy in the early afternoon and productivity is usually lower. Since 2 p.m. is our body's natural low point, players are likely to be sleepier, less alert, and slower during this natural lull. Meanwhile, the visiting teams—depending on which time zone they traveled from—are usually spared from this.

By the fourth quarter, around 2:30 p.m., my team and its fans often rally again.

Gaining a Home Time Zone Advantage

So, what happens at night? Our circadian rhythm is at its *peak* at 7–8 p.m., which is why it's called "prime time" for TV.

A 2013 study found that during football games that started at 8 p.m. or later, West Coast teams had a distinct advantage over East Coast teams, performing better during this time slot. This even matched each team's record of wins and losses.[214] In a study published in *Sports Health* in 2012, NFL data also suggest that circadian rhythms and travel across time zones may affect overall team performance.[215]

Researchers believe that the East Coast teams' biological clocks were telling them that it was already time to go to sleep, while West Coast teams were significantly more awake.[216] The effects seem to be more prominent in the later stages of the game.[217]

Can you imagine if the coaches and players were aware of this sleep phenomenon? What if they could adjust their body clocks so players don't experience being sluggish around this time? How much better could the outcome be without this third-quarter slump?

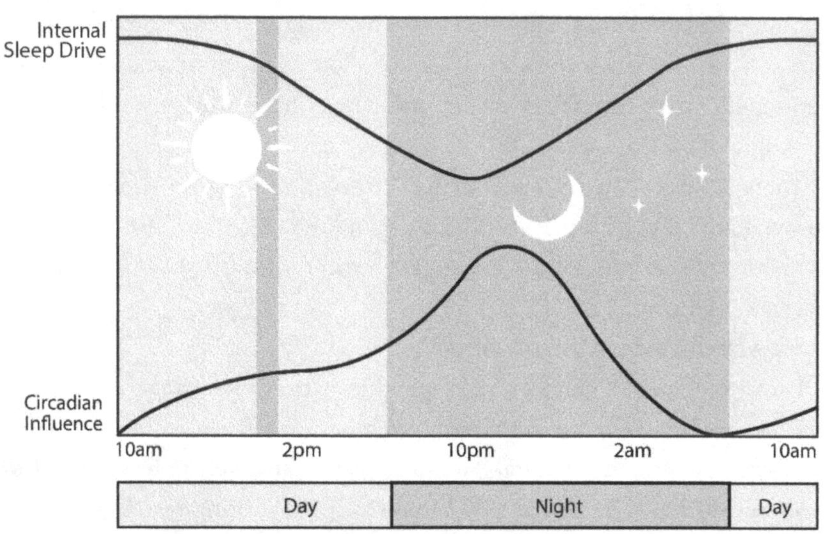

FIGURE 5. The Body's Circadian Rhythm

Your body responds to the natural influence of sunlight throughout the day. The body's internal pressure to sleep, your homeostatic pressure, begins to surge around 1:30–2 p.m. when the counterbalancing, awakening influence of the sun is not that strong. This results in early-afternoon sleepiness.

As far as my favorite team goes, I have no doubt that, with professional oversight to ensure safety, they would benefit from slightly shifting their internal clock. That way, they could actually have a "home *time zone* advantage" and be more alert during the entire game.

This can be done in a few simple ways:

- **Caffeine**: They could consume caffeine at the end of the first quarter to prevent players from being sleepy. (Caffeine is not banned by the world anti-doping agency, but it is a highly monitored substance.)
- **Diet**: A high-protein breakfast helps you to be more awake in the morning while a diet rich in carbohydrates will cause you to be sleepier. Thus, avoiding high-carb diet on the day of the game can help.
- **Exercise**: It would be a good practice to have a timed burst of strategically devised exercise at the end of the second quarter to maintain an awakened state.

But What If the Team Is Traveling?

There are a few things any team can do when traveling. (Warning: These are *not* recommended for children. Their body clocks and needs are very different from adults.)

This is similar to the strategies for dealing with jet lag.

- **Change "going to bed" time**: When changing time zones, going to bed an hour earlier or later for few days will help your body to adjust and align your circadian rhythm. (It takes a day for your body to make a one-hour change.)
  - If the team is traveling eastward and the time difference is two hours, players would need to **go to bed two hours *earlier*** for **two days** prior to travel.
  - When traveling westward and the time difference is two hours, players would need to **go to bed two hours *later*** for **two days** prior to travel date.
- **Arrive early:** Another option includes **traveling a few days earlier** and giving the athletes' bodies a chance to adjust to the local time. (If traveling from Miami to LA, for example, you'll need to arrive at least three days ahead of the game day.)
- **Avoid naps**: Surprisingly, it's better to avoid naps when traveling in and out of time zones. Naps in the new time zone can make the problem worse by preventing nighttime sleep.
- **Consider caffeine:** To maintain alertness during the day, caffeine can be used.
- **Try light-box therapy**: Another strategy is to use light-box therapy to help with adjustment of the internal clock. The light therapy can be used for 30 minutes in the morning for two days prior to travel to shift the internal clock backward, and in the evening to shift the internal clock forward.

Please note: The use of caffeine and light-box therapy should only be considered after discussing with a team medical doctor and coaching staff.

Where appropriate, college and professional athletes need to be screened for sleep disorders, specifically sleep apnea and insufficient sleep, which can have a profound impact on their performance and general health.

Athletes and coaching staff also need to be aware of the circadian influence to mitigate the symptoms for peak performance with special attention given to when the team is traveling so they can deal with time zone changes and jet lag.

As a season-ticket holder and NFL fan, I have witnessed the impact of the circadian influence on teams firsthand for many years. But this is fixable. . . and I suspect my team would win a few more games if they paid attention to this issue.

Of course, this strategy can also be used in other sports (not only for teams) as well as with travel for work or leisure.

Do Athletes Need More Sleep than Nonathletes?

Obviously, every person's sleep needs vary. That said, I generally recommend a solid seven to eight hours to my clients, particularly those who are involved in high-level sports.

Those with a later bedtime, especially younger athletes, can find this need for more sleep clashes with their training schedules—especially if they are required to work out early in the morning. But athletic accuracy—such as a quarterback passing to his receiver or a gymnast sticking their landing—improves the more sleep that a person gets.

It makes sense that athletes would want to get as much sleep as possible, yet a 2017 study conducted in South Africa showed that athletes may be getting *less* sleep than their nonathletic peers. The study included 800 elite athletes, and it found that nearly 75% slept fewer than eight hours, while 11% slept fewer than six hours at night.[218]

Some of this could be due to RLS, which makes sleep elusive and has been shown to be more common in athletes than nonathletes.[219]

The culprit is sleep-negative routines, as supported by a 2018 study that found that many elite athletes had poor sleep hygiene habits, including using devices late at night, eating heavy meals before bed, and generally shouldering a lot of stress. This study found that 41% of the 98 elite athletes surveyed could qualify as "poor sleepers," and 12% had a diagnosable sleep disorder.[220]

Understandably, many athletes also report extra difficulty falling asleep the night before a competition. Several studies have shown a direct correlation between sleep quality and sports performance and sports related injuries.[221]

Though more research into the sleep habits of athletes is needed, I'm pleased to report that a new assessment tool specifically for athletes was developed in 2020. This survey, called the **athlete sleep screening questionnaire** (ASSQ), has been designed to detect sleep disturbances and daytime dysfunction that may be unique to athletes.[222]

One study that used the ASSQ revealed that over 65% of young athletes with poor quality or duration of sleep had sport related injuries.[223]

On the flip side, when athletes get more sleep, their performance notably improves. One study found that a "1.6-hour sleep extension was associated with a 36% to 41% increase in serving accuracy" in tennis players.[224] Basketball players who increased their nightly sleep duration saw their free throw accuracy increase. Runners also logged faster sprint times after getting a longer night of sleep.[225]

This evidence shows that athletes need just as much—if not more—sleep as non-athletes. Sleep is not only essential to everyday tasks like working and studying, but also to reaching our highest athletic abilities. And athletes' muscles need more time to heal after intense physical activity.

These statistics should be an eye opener for athletes and coaches. Identifying these sleep patterns and making the necessary corrections to ensure good sleep practices is essential for optimal performance.

This is why I recommend screening athletes (whether at high school, college, or professional level) for sleep issues, and I recommend working with sports medicine clinicians, sleep specialists, and trainers to identify sleep patterns and diagnose potential sleep disorders.

When these issues are treated, athletes will have a better chance of performing at the highest level.

Naps and Sleep Debt

It was midafternoon on a Saturday, and Kristen's husband couldn't find her. After a quick search, Justin found her sitting on the bathroom floor, tears pouring down her face.

Kristen had always dreamed of being a mom, snuggling a new little person in her arms and counting fingers and toes. . . That day had finally arrived a few weeks ago with the birth of their precious newborn.

The delivery had gone well, and while Kristen knew she'd been in for some sleepless nights, she hadn't expected what it would feel like to have a colicky baby—a baby who *never* seemed to sleep.

She swaddled her and rocked her. She nursed her and put her in a swing. She rubbed her little belly and gave her warm baths. Justin played music and sang to her. They even turned the hairdryer on for white noise to soothe her.

But day after day, night after night, their sweet baby just cried and cried. Kristen knew she'd eventually grow out of it, and they were doing everything they could to comfort her in the meantime.

When Justin found his wife on the floor, he pulled her up, wrapped her in his arms, and said the sweetest words she had ever heard: "I'll take her. I think you need a nap."

No one understands the importance of naps like parents do.

Naps, short periods of sleep taken during the day, are a lifeline for new mothers, providing crucial moments of respite during the whirlwind that is early motherhood. The demands of caring for a newborn with their round-the-clock feedings and diaper changes can be physically and emotionally draining. Naps offer an opportunity for mothers to recharge both their bodies and minds. They serve as a precious window of self-care, allowing time to replenish their energy, reduce the risk of postpartum depression, and improve their overall well-being.

Naps not only enhance a mother's ability to be attentive and responsive to her baby's needs but also promote a sense of balance in her own life, reminding her that taking care of herself is an essential part of the nurturing journey she embarks upon as a new mother.

But naps are as important (or even more) for children.

When kids are little, a nap can mean the difference between a happy baby and a screaming, red-faced little monster. For young children, naps are beneficial for memory consolidation, emotional regulation, and concentration.

Though naps are not as important for learning and development as nighttime sleep is, children who napped performed better in a series of tests measuring their recall, coordination, and other measures. Naps are most important in infanthood and become more optional in the preschool years.

From the time I was little, my mom instilled the habit of afternoon naps in me, and I still encourage my family to do the same. This time coincides with the low point of the circadian rhythm, where our bodies follow the cycle of daytime and nighttime, being most alert at 7 a.m. and 7 p.m. and least alert at 2 p.m. and 2 a.m.

A short, 20–30-minute nap can be rejuvenating—some would even say *life-changing.*

Daytime Naps

Naps can be incredibly beneficial for both our physical and mental well-being. They serve to recharge and rejuvenate our bodies, allowing us to regain energy and improve our overall alertness and cognitive function.

When we engage in activities that require sustained focus and concentration, such as studying or working, our brains can become fatigued over time. A well-timed nap can help counteract this fatigue and enhance our productivity and performance.

Naps are beneficial for individuals of all ages, although the frequency and duration may vary. Young children and infants naturally require more sleep throughout the day, and regular napping is crucial for their growth and development. However, naps are not limited to the young; adults can also benefit from incorporating naps into their daily routines.

Whether you are a student, a professional, or a retiree, napping can provide an opportunity to alleviate sleep deficits, reduce stress, and enhance overall cognitive functioning, provided you don't suffer from insomnia or lack consolidated sleep at night.

The timing of a nap is important to ensure its effectiveness. It is generally recommended to *take a nap during the early afternoon*, typically between 1:30 and 3 p.m. This timeframe aligns with the body's natural dip in energy levels, often referred to as the post-lunch slump. By taking a nap during this period, we can optimize the benefits of restorative sleep without interfering with nighttime sleep.

The duration of a nap can vary depending on individual preferences and schedules, ranging from a power nap of 10–20 minutes to a longer nap of 60–90 minutes. Shorter naps are ideal for boosting alertness and combating fatigue, while longer naps can provide a more complete cycle of sleep, including both light and deep sleep stages.

Naps are valuable tools for promoting overall well-being and combating the effects of sleep deprivation. They can help improve alertness, enhance cognitive function, and reduce stress levels. Napping is beneficial for individuals of all ages, and the timing and duration of a nap should be tailored to personal preferences and schedules.

By incorporating naps into your daily routine, you can optimize your productivity, mental clarity, and overall health.

The Benefits of Naps for Adults

Children aren't the only ones who benefit from daytime naps. A recent study by University College London showed that adults who take regular naps have larger brains on average than those who didn't.[226]

Our brains shrink as we age, but those who nap were able to significantly slow this process. Researchers also noted that frequent nappers had a lower risk of cognitive decline.[227]

Many older adults have difficulty sleeping due to changes in sleep architecture that occur with age. But if you intend to add napping to your daily routine, keep the naps short.

Short naps are acceptable if they don't occur too late in the day while longer naps may compromise nighttime sleep, which is crucial for memory consolidation and cognitive health. For this reason, I recommend that older adults limit their naps to 20 minutes a day.

For most people, I recommend 20–30-minute naps, or **power naps**. This length is perfect for boosting energy and lifting mood without causing grogginess or difficulty sleeping at night. Many folks find a power nap offers a short period of rest that can enhance alertness and cognitive function, helping them feel more energized and focused throughout the day by improving focus, memory, creativity, and problem-solving skills, making power naps an effective strategy for increasing productivity.

This can be a great way to revive yourself if you've had a poor night's sleep or a particularly challenging morning and need to refresh yourself to face the rest of the day. Setting an alarm can help you make sure you don't sleep for too long and risk drowsiness upon waking.

In my career, I have used power naps effectively to survive long shifts in the ICU.

But during times when I've battled insomnia, I steered clear of naps. Likewise, I don't encourage anyone with insomnia to take naps, even short ones, as these can prevent them from having consolidated sleep at night by releasing the sleep pressure that you are trying to build for the night.

If you are a healthy sleeper, short naps are good.

A word of caution: Long naps—i.e., naps of more than one hour—could mean you could have sleep, medical, or psychological disorder. People who suffer from depression often nap a lot. If you are sleep-deprived and suffer from ISS (insufficient sleep syndrome), naps could be making up for less time spent sleeping at night and this can lead to a vicious cycle of less sleep at night and compensatory napping during the day.

Chapter 13

Sleep Treatments

7 Proven Sleep Strategies for Better Health and Happiness

Everybody needs sleep, and when life happens and you don't get the sleep you need, you are aware by now that it can have a profound impact on your heart, brain, memory, mental health, weight, sex, and cognition, among other things.

No one is immune to situations that affect our sleep quality—not even me as a sleep doctor. But I have been determined to find long-term solutions for myself and for my patients, and in these pages, I'll share those with you.

Over the years I have developed and refined several proven sleep strategies that have helped me, my family, and hundreds of patients. I believe these strategies can also help you and your family to get the best night's sleep and "sleep proof" your life.

What follows are some of my favorite and most effective sleep strategies that have helped *hundreds* of people to wean off addictive medications and maladaptive routines.

Notice that I didn't call these strategies *quick* or *easy*. Some are easier than others, but making these changes takes discipline, determination, and significant commitment. It will take at least four to six weeks before you see noticeable improvement. For some, it can even take up to six months.

Considering you may have been sleeping poorly for years, a few weeks or months of forging new rhythms is worth every ounce of effort.

The first few days will be hard, especially keeping a fixed schedule. But if you stick with the program, you'll be ecstatic at the results.

1. Create a Sleep Plan

The best sleep plan includes **a fixed sleep schedule**—*including on weekends*. The ideal sleep window for most folks is 10 p.m. to 6 a.m. Sticking to a fixed plan helps to consolidate sleep and establish a stable pattern, which will form the foundation for all the other changes you'll be making.

- If your current sleep cycle is far different from the ideal 10 p.m. to 6 a.m. schedule, use **sleep restriction**, a proven method to consolidate sleep. If you try to go to sleep at 10 p.m. but cannot fall asleep till midnight, start by going to bed around 11:30 p.m. at first, and get up at 6 a.m. Do *not* take a nap during the day. The aim is to create sleep debt, and a nap will wipe out the sleep debt.

  After at least a week of consolidated sleep with the new schedule, you can move your bedtime back by 15–30 minutes. Continue doing this until you go to bed at 10 p.m. and get a good eight hours of sleep.

  A word of caution: Sleep restriction is not advised for folks suffering from certain psychological disorders. If that's you and you want to adjust your sleep patterns, seek the guidance of your primary care physician or a sleep specialist.
- **Be strict about following your new sleep schedule.** Only alter it once you have a stable sleep pattern. *This can take several weeks.*
- **Set an alarm and get up consistently at the same time every day,** even if you didn't sleep well. Resist the temptation to hit snooze as it defeats the purpose of forging a new sleep pattern.
- Meanwhile, get to know about your sleep patterns by keeping a **Sleep Journal** (available at the back of the book, or to download at SleepFixAcademy.com) for at least two weeks. This will help you to identify any poor habits that are hindering sleep.

  The Sleep Journal will have you note what time you worked out, when you took a nap, when you drank alcohol, when you went to sleep, the number of times you woke up, what time you got up, and when you drank your first and last caffeinated drink. Also make a note of other habits to identify their impact on your sleep.

If you wear an Apple watch, Fitbit, or similar monitoring device while sleeping, you can incorporate the data these devices provide you. By observing the data, you can identify habits that need to be tweaked to create your sleep plan.

If the Sleep Journal reveals you are going to sleep at 10 p.m. and struggling to fall asleep till midnight, the common mistake most people make is to try go to sleep *earlier*. But this only worsens the problem as you'll struggle longer to fall asleep. Instead, I recommend utilizing a sleep restriction strategy.

Also do a **Sleep Assessment** (again, available at the back of the book, or to download at SleepFixAcademy.com) for a month to help you identify potential sleep disruptors that need to be addressed as well as to monitor progress.

2. Create a Sleep-Friendly Environment

Find ways to be comfortable while you're sleeping.

- **Keep your bedroom dark.** If light is entering someplace and you cannot block it, wear an eye mask. Fortunately, eye masks have come a long way. You can even get a mask that allows you to open your eyes, so it appears dark, while the mask doesn't put pressure on your eyeballs.
- **Keep your bedroom cool.** Darkness optimizes the secretion of natural melatonin, and sleep quality is better with cooler temperatures, around 65–70 degrees. If a cooler room is too cold for your partner, offer them a few extra blankets for their side of the bed!
- **Sleep in comfortable night clothes** (PJs, night shirts, or *au natural*). If you have night sweats, wear breathable fabrics that will help wick away any moisture.
- **Use a weighted blanket** to provide extra heaviness and coziness.
- **Eliminate distracting noises.** If ambient noises tend to wake you up, get a **white noise machine** or wear comfortable **earplugs**.
- **Try aroma therapy**. Lavender, in particular, can have a soothing effect.
- **Follow your doctor-prescribed sleep instructions.** If you have sleep apnea, get a **CPAP** machine—*and use it, even if you find it to be uncomfortable in the beginning!*

3. Eliminate (or Minimize) Your Electronics

The bedroom should only be for sex and sleep, not for phones, tablets, and laptop computers.

Light emitted by electronics signals to the brain to be awake. As a result, the brain doesn't secrete melatonin, which is needed to sleep. Beyond that, using technology invokes the thought process, making it harder to shut off our minds and drift off. Plus, some apps can also be extremely addictive. You may log in to check something and find yourself an hour or two later still scrolling or playing games.

- **Keep your eyes off screens.** For *at least an hour* prior to going to sleep, **do not watch television or use electronics**—including cell phones or tablets (iPads). There are several reasons to practice this boundary.
- **Remove the TV from your bedroom.** Not only are the bright lights confusing to your body's natural rhythm, but news programs containing negative or unsettling information, for example, can also directly affect your sleep.
- **Remove the clock from the bedroom.** It's normal to sometimes wake up in the middle of the night. But when you look at the clock and see the time—for example, noticing that it is 3 a.m.—it creates an awakening response. (*I have only slept three hours!* or *I must wake up soon. . .*) which only makes it harder to fall back to sleep.
- **Remove your phone from the bedroom.** This helps you to break the habits of random scrolling and reaching for your phone when you wake up.
- **Set an alarm to wake up at the same time every morning.** If your alarm is on your phone, even better. It would mean you'd have to get up and leave the room to turn off the alarm.

A word about phone addiction: If you struggle with phone addiction, all the more reason to remove the phone from your bedroom and turn off all notifications during your sleep window. Concerned about not hearing the phone in the event of an emergency? Turn on the setting that allows calls to go through from certain phone numbers if someone calls you quickly two times in a row.

4. Calm Your Body

Signal to your body that it's time to sleep.

- **Don't exercise too late.** Exercise releases endorphins, which act as a stimulant, affecting sleep quality. For at least four hours before bedtime, don't engage in heavy exercise. Gentle exercise, like taking a leisurely walk or stretching promotes healthy sleep.

- **Avoid caffeinated products** at least six hours prior to going to sleep. Caffeine typically lingers in the body for 5–6 hours, but for some folks, the effects can linger up to 10 or 12 hours. I advise my clients not to have any caffeinated products after 1 p.m.
- **Don't drink excessive alcohol.** The sedative properties of alcohol are well known, but alcohol metabolizes into acetaldehyde within 3–4 hours, causing frequent awakenings and confusion. Plus, alcohol is a diuretic and can result in you having to use the restroom at night.

  Enjoying a glass of wine or beer with others is typically fine, but if you start relying on alcohol to go to sleep, that's a sign of an unhealthy dependence.
- **Avoid eating a large meal** less than two hours prior to going to sleep. Also avoid spicy, fatty, and carb-heavy foods at night.
- **Hydrate throughout the day**, then limit water intake starting around 8 p.m. This can help you avoid waking up to use the restroom in the middle of the night.
- **Practice relaxing your body** through belly breathing, also called diaphragmatic breathing.[228] Once in bed, place one hand on your chest and one on your belly. Relax. Breathe in slowly through your nose. Instead of feeling your chest rise, follow the air and pay attention to fill your belly. Exhale slowly as your chest remains still. Repeat these slow and even breaths.
- **Complete a body scan.** Another relaxing practice you can do in bed is progressive muscle relaxation. Starting at the top of your body, scan the muscles one area at a time for any tension, then release the tension.

  If you start at the top of your body, for example, scan your facial muscles for tension to release—the muscles of your forehead, around the eyes and nose, the cheeks and jaw—then the muscles at the back of your neck, the front of your neck, the shoulders. Continue all the way down to your feet, each time releasing any tension you notice.

5. Calm Your Mind

Now that your body is relaxed, you can relax your mind by changing your mental focus to and creating a sleep state.

- **Avoid cognitively challenging activities near bedtime.** Do not indulge in physical or cognitive activity like cleaning, paying bills, answering emails, or using your electronic gadgets close to bedtime.

- **Focus on your breath.** Dr. Andrew Weil developed a breathing method that forces the mind and body to focus on regulating the breath rather than replaying your worries when you lie down at night. Sit comfortably or lie down, then use the 4–7–8 technique.

  Before starting the breathing pattern, adopt a comfortable sitting position, then place the tip of the tongue right behind the top front teeth. Next, try the following breathing pattern:

  - Empty the lungs of air.
  - Breath in quietly through the nose for **four** seconds.
  - Hold your breath for a count of **seven** seconds.
  - With pursed lips, exhale forcefully through the mouth for **eight** seconds, making a "whoosh" sound.
  - Repeat the cycle up to four times.

  You may feel lightheaded after doing this for the first few times. Therefore, it is advisable to try this technique when sitting or lying down to prevent dizziness or falls. As long as you maintain the correct ratio, you may notice benefits after several days or weeks of doing 4–7–8 breathing consistently one to two times a day.[229]

- **Practice yogic sleep.** One ancient practice that has risen in popularity of late to treat insomnia is yoga *nidra*. There are several types of yoga which all focus on body posture and breathing. But yoga *nidra*, otherwise known as yogic sleep, focuses on the meditative aspect.

  Nidra is derived from Sanskrit word meaning a state of nothingness equivalent to deep sleep. This practice is believed to help calm the nervous system, secrete melatonin, and combat anxiety. The best part is that this practice does not need an instructor. You can do this in the comfort of your own home.

  Simply lie on your back with your arms to the side in what is called the *savasana* (corpse pose) and be comfortable. Your legs should be about 30 degrees apart, arms about 45 degrees away from the sides of the body. You can use a pillow to support your neck if you prefer.

  Allow up to a minute to settle your body into its laying position. As you start to relax, think positive thoughts as you ease into a restful state. Observe your breath. Do not attempt to control the breath, neither the amount of air taken in or out nor in the length of the breath in or out.

  Repeat this daily for 15–20 minutes as you get ready for sleep.

- **Focus on prayer.** Sometimes it's important to just give things over to a Higher Power, especially when we're trying to sleep and our mind is racing out of control. Reciting prayers and verses can help you focus your mind outside yourself as you try and sleep.
- **Practice Vivid Imagination®**. I also recommend a technique I have developed called Vivid Imagination® to help you ease into sleep.

  This is a process by which you start engaging your imagination to create a story. You can even start by reading a novel or thinking of a show you have watched earlier.

  Form your own ideas about what happens in the next chapter or episode and try to guess how the story will end. Losing yourself in a story makes it easy to drift off to sleep, and if you wake up in the middle of the night, you can simply continue where you left off.
- **What about when you wake up?** If you do wake up in the middle of the night for any reason like needing to go to the restroom, **preserve the delicate semi-sleep state** and get back to bed as quickly and as gently as possible.

  Do not do anything stimulating like looking at the clock or phone, cleaning, paying bills, or turning on the TV. This can lead to awakenings and the inability to go back to sleep. Seeing the time can also increase your anxiety and prevent you from sleeping.

  If you wake up and cannot get back to sleep, leave the bedroom. Do something simple but do *not* increase cognitive or physical activity, e.g., read a novel (physical book, not on a screen), knit, journal, or practice breathing techniques. But don't do so in bed. Your bed is for sleeping. After 30 minutes, go back to bed.

  Even if you still don't sleep well for the rest of the night, still *get up at the fixed time*. This is the only way to consolidate sleep.

6. Schedule Worry Time

In my first year of starting my private practice, I used to constantly worry about the issues of the day once I went to bed. This was affecting my quality of sleep. I started working on a method by having a designated time in the evening to problem solve.

This may seem strange, but if you struggle with anxiety or racing thoughts—whether on occasion or all the time—downloading your thoughts before you try and go to sleep may be a great solution. Do this 2–3 hours before heading to your bedroom.

- **Take a few minutes to think about the persisting issues on your mind**. These could be decisions you have to make, concerns about family, work, bills, taxes, disagreements, politics—whatever weighs on your mind.
- **Grab a journal and write it all down.** This relieves the pressure to keep it all in your head. If feasible, also think of ways to resolve these worries. *Do not take these thoughts to your bedroom or try to resolve them while in bed.*
- If, after finishing your list, you still feel concerned, **add the item to the next day's to-do list**. But even if you cannot think of a solution, simply seeing it in writing will help you put it aside as you go to sleep, knowing you can tackle it at another time. And as pointed out earlier, you may want to release the concern through prayer.

7. Simplify Your Sleep Routine

Your bedtime routines should be simple and few. Adding too many routines and making going to bed too complicated only keeps your mind going, causing your sleep plan to backfire. To get back to sleeping like a baby, gently turn off your revved-up mind (and body) in a thoughtful and systemic manner. The process of initiating sleep should be as simple as 1-2-3.

If you want a routine to follow every night, use only the simplest sleep-positive routines. These can include:

- sticking to a fixed schedule,
- playing soothing music (but don't reintroduce the temptation of bringing your phone to bed!) or having soothing white noise as a background noise, and
- wearing an eye mask.

Of all the sleep strategies mentioned, the key is *simplification* to calm the mind and body.

If you can follow these proven methods, it can get you back on the right track and enjoy the benefits of refreshing sleep for the rest of your life.

And if you sleep well, you can feel better, be more successful, and live a much happier life.

Cognitive Behavioral Therapy for Insomnia

In addition to these sleep strategies, if you still struggle to sleep, a well-recognized and scientifically proven method for treating many forms of insomnia is CBT-I, as mentioned before.

In fact, the evidence for CBT-I's effectiveness is overwhelming, and in 2016, the American College of Physicians made a landmark recommendation that CBT-I should be the first line of treatment for people with chronic insomnia.[230]

CBT-I is based on the principle that psychological problems are caused, at least in part, by our thought processes. The theory goes, if we can fix the thought process, we can fix our mood and behavior.

CBT-I is performed best by mental health professionals who are experts in this field.

The top five guidelines for CBT-I include **sleep restriction** to consolidate sleep. Once sleep hygiene and sleep restriction are established, the next phase of improving sleep is to work on **stimulus control**, i.e., identifying the stimulus that is causing insomnia. Once stimuli have been removed, you'll focus on **relaxation therapy** to engage your body's natural relaxation response. This is followed by **visualization** exercises, using mental images to create a sense of well-being in the body. Finally, **body scans** are used as a meditative practice to focus inward and release any stress from the day.

Medications to Treat Insomnia

Multiple sleeping aids—from over-the-counter options to various prescription medications—have entered the market over the years. Though they may help for a night or two, none of these medications are effective in the long term. In fact, the side effects can be devastating if used for too long, because the more a person uses them to induce sleep, the more they come to rely on them.

The side effects of sleeping pills can last over 12 hours, causing folks to feel groggy the next morning, needing stimulants to combat the effects of the sleep medication and get them through the day.

My ultimate treatment goal is to help people taper off and wean them from their sleep medications. In fact, I have weaned several hundred people from multiple sleeping aids over my years in practice.

As a physician, I also know that that there is a group of people who, due to specific conditions, require medications to help them be functional in their daily life. I only prescribe sleep medications in such cases, and once the underlying issues have been addressed, I frequently reassess the need for continued need for medications.

The group of medications that typically treat insomnia are called hypnotics. They are divided into two categories: over-the-counter medications and prescription medications.

Popular over-the-counter medications for sleep are melatonin, acetaminophen PM, and diphenhydramine. There are also many helpful over-the-counter supplements available that could help with sleep, including magnesium, valerian root, ashwagandha, and tryptophan sleep aid.

The most prescribed hypnotic medications are zolpidem, eszopiclone, zaleplon, alprazolam, and diazepam. These medications augment the GABA receptors in the brain that induce sleep. But these receptors are present in various parts of the brain, and when these medications are taken, they affect multiple parts of the brain, causing unwanted side effects like dizziness, persistence of sleepiness during the day, risk of developing a tolerance, abuse, and medication dependence.

People on these medications are also at risk for falls, and when these medications are combined with alcohol, they can have even more deleterious consequences. Long-term usage can cause memory and cognitive issues; however, this damage could be halted if the person stops taking these medications. Some antidepressants like trazadone and doxepin are commonly used to treat insomnia with varying success.

While prescriptions for sleep have typically been limited to these GABA drugs, a new class of medicine is creating a lot of enthusiasm in the sleep medicine community. These new medications focus on the specific receptors that cause the awakenings that trigger insomnia. This group of new medications is called DORAs (dual orexin receptor antagonists) and include daridorexant, suvorexant, and lemborexant.

Normally in insomnia, the awakenings are caused by the orexin receptors that secrete wakefulness-stimulating hormones in the brain (like histamine, dopamine, and norepinephrine) which make us feel alert, making it difficult to fall back asleep.

DORAs selectively block the orexin receptors and, therefore, can prevent the secretion of these wakefulness-promoting hormones.

Among the available DORAs in the market, Quvivig® (daridorexant)[231] has the shortest half-life of eight hours. Hence, it correlates well with sleep time and could result in less grogginess the next morning.

A word of caution: The American Academy of Sleep Medicine does not recommend use of prescription medication sedatives for more than six months. For this reason, I try to see my clients every few months to re-evaluate their treatment.

Chapter 14

Conclusion

When the Smith family came to the sleep clinic, it didn't take long to discover that they had been living under the heavy cloud of unhappiness for quite some time.

Ronald, Jemila, and Tyrone sat in the waiting room looking tired and disconnected, Ronald on one side of the room, Jamila, on the other, and Tyrone in the middle, focused on his phone.

It is unusual for me to see an entire family, but the Smiths were *all* having sleep issues.

Tyrone was 16 years old with dreams of becoming a professional golfer. However, he had been having trouble sleeping for the past few months since his breakup with his longtime girlfriend. His mom was very concerned as she said his once cheerful demeanor had faded, and he had lost interest in golf. (He had loved golf since he was little and had seen Tiger Woods play.)

Tyrone said he just didn't care anymore and didn't have the energy to play golf.

Jemila was visibly distressed about her son. She said he had always been a jovial, happy-go-lucky kid who took great pleasure in being out on the golf course. He was the bright spot in her family, and to see him like this was heart wrenching.

Jemila was 51 and was peri-menopausal, and her sleep was affected by hot flashes at night. Plus, she was bothered by Ronald's snoring, so much so that they had been sleeping separately—i.e., having a sleep divorce. Ronald was sleeping in his recliner or on the couch most nights.

Ronald had just turned 50 and had been snoring loudly for over five years. He said his snoring never bothered *him*. He admitted, though, that his energy level was not what it used to be, his sex life was nonexistent, and he was scared of falling asleep at the wheel while driving to work.

During a recent executive physical, his lab testing revealed he had high blood pressure and his testosterone was low. His manager at work had even remarked during his performance evaluation that Ronald seemed to be less attentive at work, and he inquired to see if there was a problem at home.

This family was struggling and unhappy for many reasons, but the underlying reason for all of them was poor sleep.

They had all completed a Sleep Journal and Sleep Assessment prior to the appointment, and I found that Tyrone was only averaging around six hours of sleep each night, while Jemila was getting around 5–6 hours a night, and Ronald 7 hours.

During the consultation, it was evident that Tyrone was sleeping poorly after his breakup and had fallen into depression.

With help from a psychiatric colleague of mine, Tyrone was able to deal with his depression. He implemented the *7 Proven Sleep Strategies*, starting by following a strict sleep schedule. He was able to sleep better. His broken heart also started to mend. Over time, he was back playing golf and his overall quality of life had improved.

I referred Jemila to an OB/GYN who specialized in hormone replacement therapy for her menopause symptoms. As her hormone issues got addressed and as her sleep improved, her spirits lifted, and she said she felt like a new person.

Ronald, after doing an in-home sleep study, had evidence of severe sleep apnea, and he finally started to understand the deeper implications of his sleep issues.

He began using a CPAP, he and Jemila were reunited in the bedroom, and their intimacy improved.

Their family struggles were interconnected, and addressing their sleep issues was, in this case, the key to them all feeling better.

A study published in 2018 revealed how good sleep can positively affect how one feels about life,[232] and the Smiths' story is a testament to this transformative power of good sleep. Their story is a reminder that when we take care of our sleep, we pave the way for a more fulfilling and happier life.

Everyone is vulnerable to having sleeping issues at some time or another because, as we all know, "life happens."

But the question is: are your sleep issues interfering in your life or in the life of someone you love?

When we can't sleep, we can usually feel the toll that lack of sleep has on our mind and our body. We also sense the implications for our health, productivity, and how we enjoy life.

And for many people—particularly when it comes to sleep apnea—the sound of loud snoring can be equally as disruptive to *someone else's sleep*. Meanwhile, we can be blissfully unaware of the toll it is taking on our mind and body.

By now I hope you have come to realize that there truly are options when it comes to sleeping better and feeling better. And when we feel better, we become happier in all areas of life.

Remember, if you're "tired of being tired," you're not alone.

There are many things you can do on your own to help you sleep. If you follow the *7 Proven Sleep Strategies*, relief may not happen overnight, but consistently using these strategies will help you get a better sleep.

But if you're still struggling, or if you're lovingly being told you need to get help, there are also many options available through a sleep doctor that can make a difference in the quantity and *quality* of the sleep you get.

It is my heartfelt hope that you understand that deep, restful, restorative sleep is possible.

Your journey to better health begins tonight. May you sleep better, be more productive, and live a happier—and less tired—life.

About the Author

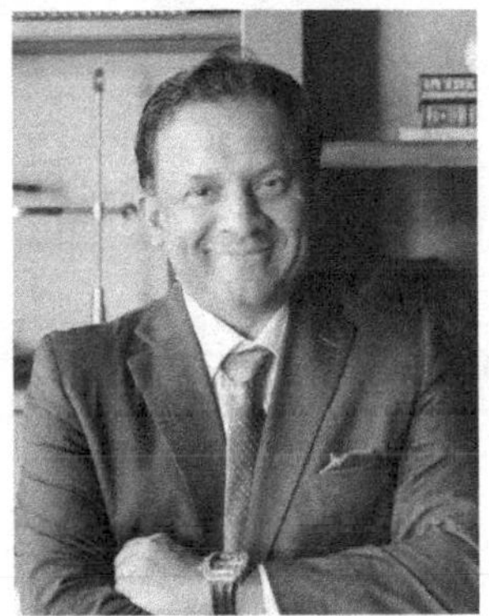

Dr. Bijoy E. John is a board-certified physician and practicing sleep specialist currently in private practice. He has over 25 years of experience in pulmonary medicine, critical care, and sleep medicine, treating children and adults with various sleep disorders. He is the Founder and Medical Director of Sleep Wellness Clinics of America PLLC in Brentwood, TN and Sleep Fix Academy LLC.

Dr. John is a member of American College of Physicians, American Medical Association, the American College of Chest Physicians, and the American Academy of Sleep Medicine. He was awarded the Top 100 Physicians in Nashville for 2022 (*My Nashville Magazine*) and the top Sleep Specialist award several years in a row (2015–2020) by his peers and patients (*Nashville Lifestyles Magazine*). His Tennessee State Respiratory Care Program achieved top respiratory therapy department recognition in the state during his tenure as Medical Director (2001–2010).

In 2001, Dr. John achieved board certification in four specialties in medicine: internal medicine, pulmonary diseases, critical care medicine, and sleep medicine. As his private practice grew, he felt the patients with sleep problems were neglected as the issues were non-emergencies compared to patients who had pulmonary, cardiac, or neurological issues. He decided to focus on this underserved area and started his own clinic so he could reach a wider audience and spread the word of hope for anyone who struggles with sleep issues.

Dr. John has been married to his wife, Dotty, for more than 30 years, and they have two children, Brandon and Rachael. They live in Brentwood, TN. In his spare time, Dr. John enjoys golfing, traveling, writing, playing tennis, and working on his coral reef aquarium.

Contact Dr. John at:

Bijoy E. John MD, FCCP
1612 Westgate Circle, Suite 210
Brentwood, TN 37027

You can also connect with Dr. John at:

SleepWellnessInfo.com
SleepFixAcademy.com
DrSleepFix@gmail.com

And be sure to follow Dr. John:

Instagram (Dr.SleepFix),
Facebook (DrSleepFix and SleepFixAcademy), and
TikTok (@Dr.SleepFix).
You can also find him on LinkedIn.com/in/dr-sleepfix/ and
LinkedIn.com/company/sleep-fix-academy.

Visit SleepFixAcadamy.com to download the Sleep Journal and Sleep Assessment.

About the Sleep Wellness Clinics of America and Sleep Fix Academy

Sleep Wellness Clinics of America (SWCA) led by Dr. Bijoy E. John, is a private clinic dedicated to the diagnosis and treatment of various sleep disorders. With over 25 years of experience in this field, Dr. John's focus is to treat patients with the utmost care, offering the latest technology with emphasis on home diagnosis and offering one-stop care. SWCA offers the full range of sleep-medicine services, including diagnostic and therapeutic interventions, second opinions, compliance monitoring, and more.

Sleep Fix Academy (SleepFixAcademy.com) is an online resource to access podcasts, online courses, books, the Sleep Journal, Sleep Assessment, and more.

Resources

Sleep Journal

Instructions

Note what might be impacting your sleep by tracking events from noon to noon.

1. Indicate the main focus of your day—if you're at work, school, at home, on vacation, or on a day off.
2. At various hours throughout the day, indicate with a C when you consume caffeinated drinks, A if you consume alcohol, E if you exercise, N for a nap, and S for when you go to bed.
3. Shade the boxes for the hours you believe you were asleep.

Sleep Assessment

Instructions

Your sleep assessment score (SAS) is a self-reported score based on your sleep quality in a week, tracked for one month.

- Please rate yourself in each of the areas listed on a scale of 0–3.
- After a month, add up your score.
- If your total SAS is more than 6, your sleep quality is poor and you need to consult with your primary care physician.

SLEEP JOURNAL

	Date	Day	Focus	Noon	1 p.m.	2 p.m.	3 p.m.	4 p.m.	5 p.m.	6 p.m.	7 p.m.	8 p.m.	9 p.m.	10 p.m.	11 p.m.	Midnight	1 a.m.	2 a.m.	3 a.m.	4 a.m.	5 a.m.	6 a.m.	7 a.m.	8 a.m.	9 a.m.	10 a.m.	11 a.m.
Ex.	3/2	Mo	Work		E		N			A				S									C				

SLEEP ASSESSMENT

CIRCLE ONE

0 = 0 Times per week   1= 1 Time per week   2=2 Times per week   3=3+ Times per week

	Week 1	Week 2	Week 3	Week 4	
Time to fall asleep > 30 minutes	0 1 2 3	0 1 2 3	0 1 2 3	0 1 2 3	
Woke up at night	0 1 2 3	0 1 2 3	0 1 2 3	0 1 2 3	
Snored	0 1 2 3	0 1 2 3	0 1 2 3	0 1 2 3	
Partner/spouse noticed I stopped breathing in my sleep	0 1 2 3	0 1 2 3	0 1 2 3	0 1 2 3	
Felt hot or cold at night	0 1 2 3	0 1 2 3	0 1 2 3	0 1 2 3	
Got up to use the restroom	0 1 2 3	0 1 2 3	0 1 2 3	0 1 2 3	
Pain affected my sleep	0 1 2 3	0 1 2 3	0 1 2 3	0 1 2 3	
Had shortness of breath at night	0 1 2 3	0 1 2 3	0 1 2 3	0 1 2 3	
Took sleeping pills	0 1 2 3	0 1 2 3	0 1 2 3	0 1 2 3	
Was tired during the day	0 1 2 3	0 1 2 3	0 1 2 3	0 1 2 3	**Full Month Total**
Total					

Recommendations

The American Academy of Sleep Medicine | AASM.org

The American Board of Sleep Medicine | ABSM.org

The Sleep Foundation | SleepFoundation.org

The National Institute of Health | NIH.gov

The Centers for Disease Control and Prevention | CDC.gov

Sleep Wellness Clinics of America | SleepWellnessInfo.com

Sleep Fix Academy | SleepFixAcademy.com

Glossary

AHI apnea hypopnea index
ASPS advanced sleep phase syndrome
CBT cognitive behavioral therapy
CBT-I cognitive behavioral therapy for insomnia
COMISA comorbid insomnia and sleep apnea
COPD chronic obstructive pulmonary disorder, or emphysema
CPAP continuous positive airway pressure
DSPS delayed sleep phase disorder
GABA gamma-aminobutyric acid
GERD gastroesophageal reflux disease
HGH human growth hormone
IH idiopathic hypersomnia
NES nocturnal eating syndrome
OSA obstructive sleep apnea
PLMD periodic limb movement disorder
REM rapid eye movement
RBD REM behavior disorder
RLS restless leg syndrome
SCN suprachiasmatic nucleus, or internal clock
SRED sleep-related eating disorder
SSRIs selective serotonin reuptake inhibitors
SWSD shift work sleep disorder

Endnotes

Chapter 2: Desperate for Sleep

1 "Americans Feel Sleepy 3 Days a Week, With Impacts on Activities, Mood & Acuity." Sleep in America Poll, National Sleep Foundation. thensf.org/wp-content/uploads/2020/03/SIA-2020-Report.pdf.

2 "Obstructive Sleep Apnea." Johns Hopkins Medicine. hopkinsmedicine.org/health/conditions-and-diseases/obstructive-sleep-apnea.

3 Clementi, M. "Your Child's Mental Health: Why Does Sleep Matter?" Texas Children's Hospital. texaschildrens.org/blog/2016/05/your-child's-mental-health-why-does-sleep-matter.

4 National Blood, Heart, and Lung Institute. "Why Is Sleep Important?" nhlbi.nih.gov/node/4605

5 "What Happens When You Sleep?" Sleep Foundation. sleepfoundation.org/how-sleep-works/what-happens-when-you-sleep.

6 "REM Sleep Behavior Disorder." Mayo Clinic. mayoclinic.org/diseases-conditions/rem-sleep-behavior-disorder/symptoms-causes/syc-20352920.

7 Howley, E. K. and Miller, A. M. "Are Energy Drinks Really That Bad?" *U.S. News Health*. health.usnews.com/wellness/fitness/energy-drinks.

8 Knutsson, A. "Shift Work and Coronary Heart Disease." *Scandinavian Journal of Social Medicine*. 44, 1989: 1–36. pubmed.ncbi.nlm.nih.gov/2683043/.

9 Jehan, S., et al. "Shift Work and Sleep: Medical Implications and Management," *Sleep Medicine and Disorders: International Journal.* 1 (2) October 2017. ncbi.nlm.nih.gov/pmc/articles/PMC5836745/.

10 Elon Musk Reveals His Knowledge on Aliens, Challenges Putin to UFC, and Predicts WW3." *Full Send Podcast.* Published August 4, 2022. youtube.com/watch?v=fXS_gkWAIs0

11 Clifford, C. "I Need to Figure Out How to Be Better…" cnbc.com. Published April 13, 2016. cnbc.com/2018/04/13/elon-musk-talks-to-gayle-king-about-meeting-tesla-goals.html

12 Mejia, Z. "Elon Musk Sleeps Under His Desk …" cnbc.com. Published July 2, 2018. cnbc.com/2018/06/29/elon-musk-sleeps-under-a-desk-even-after-youtuber-crowdfunded-a-couch.html

13 Suni, E. "Sleep Statistics," Sleep Foundation, sleepfoundation.org/how-sleep-works/sleep-facts-statistics.

14 Dopheide, J. A. "Insomnia Overview: Epidemiology, Pathophysiology, Diagnosis and Monitoring, and Nonpharmacologic Therapy." The *American Journal of Managed Care.* Apr 12, 2020: S76–S84.

Chapter 3: Sleep Issues

15 Roth, T. "Comorbid Insomnia: Current Directions and Future Challenges." *The American Journal of Managed Care.* 15, no. 1, March 2009: S6-S13, ajmc.com/view/a228_09feb_roth_s6tos13.

16 Grandner, M. A., et al. "Mortality Associated with Short Sleep Duration: The Evidence, The Possible Mechanisms, and the Future," *Sleep Medicine Reviews.* 14 (3) June 2010: 191–203.

17 Craik, K. "The 17th Century Guide to Sleep," History Today. historytoday.com/miscellanies/17th-century-guide-sleep.

18 Dopheide, J. A. "Insomnia Overview: Epidemiology, Pathophysiology, Diagnosis and Monitoring, and Nonpharmacologic Therapy." *The American Journal of Managed Care.* 26 (4) April 2020: S76–S84.

19 "Americans Feel Sleepy 3 Days a Week with Impacts on Activities, Mood, and Acuity." Sleep in America Poll 2020. National Sleep Foundation, Langer Research Associates. thensf.org/wp-content/uploads/2020/03/SIA-2020-Report.pdf.

20 Liu, Y., et al. "Prevalence of Healthy Sleep Duration Among Adults—United States, 2014," *Morbid and Mortality Weekly Report.* 65 (6) February 2016: 137–141.

21 Dopheide, J. A. "Insomnia Overview: Epidemiology, Pathophysiology, Diagnosis and Monitoring, and Nonpharmacologic Therapy." *The American Journal of Managed Care.* 26 (4) April 2020: S76–S84.
22 McNab, R. "Sweet Dreams More Important Than You Might Think." *The Joplin Globe*. Published March 17, 2023. joplinglobe.com.
23 "What to Do If You Struggle With insomnia." CareNow® Urgent Care. Published May 4, 2022. carenow.com/blog/entry/what-to-do-if-you-struggle-with-insomnia.
24 "Impact of the DSM-IV to DSM-5 Changes on the National Survey on Drug Use and Health." *National Library of Medicine*. Substance Abuse and Mental Health Services Administration, Rockville, MD. June 2016. ncbi.nlm.nih.gov/books/NBK519704/table/ch3.t36/.
25 Ji X., et al, *Sleep Health*. 5 (4) 2019: 376–381.
26 American Psychiatric Association, *Diagnostic and Statistical Manual of Mental Disorders, 5th Ed.* Washington, DC: American Psychiatric Association; 2013.
27 "The State of Sleep Health in America." Sleep Health. sleephealth.org/sleep-health/the-state-of-sleephealth-in-america/.
28 "New Campaign to Raise Awareness that Sleep Apnea Is 'More than a Snore,'" *American Academy of Sleep Medicine*. February 6, 2023. aasm.org/new-campaign-to-raise-awareness-that-sleep-apnea-is-more-than-a-snore/.
29 "Widow of NFL Legend Reggie White Promotes Awareness of Sleep Disorders," WCNC.com, November 7, 2011. wcnc.com/article/news/local/widow-of-nfl-legend-reggie-white-promotes-awareness-of-sleep-disorders/275-373933617.
30 "Bappi Lahiri Passes Away: Disco King of Bollywood Dies at 69," *The Indian Express*, 16 February 2022.
31 Young, T. et al. "Menopausal Status and Sleep-Disordered Breathing in the Wisconsin Sleep Cohort Study." *American Journal of Respiratory and Critical Care Medicine.* 167 (9) 2003: 1181–1185.
32 Leung, W. B. et al. "The Prevalence and Severity of Obstructive Sleep Apnea in Severe Obesity: The Impact of Ethnicity." *Journal of Clinical Sleep Medicine.* 9 (9). September 2013.
33 Pranathiageswaran, S. et al. "The Influence of Race on the Severity of Sleep Disordered Breathing." *Journal of Clinical Sleep Medicine.* 9 (4). April 2013.
34 Torberg, L. "Mayo Clinic Q and A: Neck Size One Risk Factor for Obstructive Sleep Apnea," Mayo Clinic News Network. June 20, 2015. newsnetwork.

mayoclinic.org/discussion/mayo-clinic-q-and-a-neck-size-one-risk-factor-for-obstructive-sleep-apnea.

35 Findley, L. J., et al. "Cognitive Impairment in Patients with Obstructive Sleep Apnea and Associated Hypoxemia," *Chest.* 90 (5) November 1986: 686–690. sciencedirect.com/science/article/abs/pii/S0012369215437821.

36 Lee, M., et al. "Association of Obstructive Sleep Apnea with White Matter Integrity and Cognitive Performance Over a 4-Year Period in Middle to Late Adulthood," *JAMA Network Open.* 5 (7) 2022. ncbi.nlm.nih.gov/pmc/articles/PMC8673645/

37 Medic, G., et al. "Short-and Long-Term Health Consequences of Sleep Disruption," *Nature and Science of Sleep.* (9) May 2017: 151–161.

38 Lee, M., et al. "Association of Obstructive Sleep Apnea with White Matter Integrity and Cognitive Performance Over a 4-Year Period in Middle to Late Adulthood." *JAMA Network Open.* 5 (7) 2022.

39 Sahib, A., et. al. "Relationships between Brain Tissue Damage, Oxygen Desaturation, and Disease Severity in Obstructive Sleep Apnea Evaluated by Diffusion Tensor Imaging." *Journal of Sleep Medicine.* 18 (12) 2022.

40 Lim, Z.W., et al. "Obstructive Sleep Apnea Increases Risk of Female Infertility: A 14-year Nationwide Population-based Study." *PLoS One.* Published only December 15, 2021. 16 (12).

41 Bahammam, A. "Obstructive Sleep Apnea: From Simple Upper Airway Obstruction to Systemic Inflammation," *Annals of Saudi Medicine.* 31 (1) January–February 2011: 1–2. ncbi.nlm.nih.gov/pmc/articles/PMC3101717.

42 Do Vale Cardoso Lopes, T., et al. "Eating Late Negatively Affects Sleep Pattern and Apnea Severity in Individuals with Sleep Apnea," *Journal of Clinical Sleep Medicine.* 15 (03) March 2019: 383–392.

43 For the sake of transparency, I have given presentations on behalf of Signifier Medical Technologies, the makers of eXciteOSA.

44 Nokes, B., et al. "The Impact of Daytime Transoral Neuromuscular Stimulation on Upper Airway Physiology: A Mechanistic Clinical Investigtion." pubmed. ncbi.nlm.nih.gov/35748091/.

45 Newsom, R. "Cataplexy," Sleep Foundation. Last modified March 21, 2023. sleepfoundation.org/physical-health/cataplexy.

46 Mayo Clinic. "Narcolepsy." Published January 14, 2023. mayoclinic.org/diseases-conditions/narcolepsy/symptoms-causes/syc-20375497.

47 Tyree, S. M., et al. "Hypocretin as a Hub for Arousal and Motivation," *Frontiers in Neurology.* 9 (413) June 2018: 1664–2295.

48 Thannickal, T. C., et al. "Localized Loss of Hypocretin (Orexin) Cells in Narcolepsy Without Cataplexy," *Sleep.* 32 (8) August 2009: 993–998.

49 Todman, D. "Narcolepsy: A Historical Review," *The Internet Journal of Neurology.* 9 (2) 2007. print.ispub.com/api/0/ispub-article/7361.

50 Sunset Sleep Diagnostics. "Narcolepsy and Cataplexy." Published March 14, 2014. sunsetsleepdiagnostics.com/features/narcolepsy-and-cataplexy/.

51 Trotti, L. M. "Idiopathic Hypersomnia: Does First to Approval Mean First-Line Treatment?" *The Lancet Neurology.* 21 (1) January 2022: 25–26.

52 Sawanyawisuth, K., et al. "Ethnic Differences in the Prevalence and Predictors of Restless Legs Syndrome between Hispanics of Mexican Descent and Non-Hispanic Whites in San Diego County: A Population-Based Study" Published January 15, 2013. pubmed.ncbi.nlm.nih.gov/23319904/.

53 Schenck, C. H., et al. "Chronic Behavioral Disorders of Human REM Sleep: A New Category of Parasomnia" *Sleep.* 1986, 9: 293–308.

54 Iranzo, A., et al. "Rapid-eye-movement Sleep Behavior Disorder as an Early Marker for a Neurodegenerative Disorder: A Descriptive Study. *The Lancet Neurology.* Vol 5, Issue 7, July 2006: 572–577.

55 Silva Brito, R., et al. "Prevalence of Insomnia in Shift Workers: A Systematic Review," *Sleep Science (Sao Paulo, Brazil).* 14 (1) 2021: 47–54. pubmed.ncbi.nlm.nih.gov/34104337/.

56 Manfredini R., et al. "Daylight Saving Time and Acute Myocardial Infarction: A Meta-analysis." *Journal of Clinical Medicine.* 8 (3). March 2019: 404. pubmed.ncbi.nlm.nih.gov/30909587/.

57 Chudow, J.J., et al. "Changes in Atrial Fibrillation Admissions Following Daylight Saving Time Transitions. *Sleep Medicine.* (69) May 2020:155–158. pubmed.ncbi.nlm.nih.gov/32088351/.

Chapter 4: Sleep and the Body

58 Dawson, D. and Reid, K. "Fatigue, Alcohol and Performance Impairment," *Nature.* 388, (6639) February 2023: 235–237.

59 Williamson, M. and Feyer, A. "Moderate Sleep Deprivation Produces Impairments in Cognitive and Motor Performance Equivalent to Legally Prescribed Levels of Alcohol Intoxication," *Occupational and Environmental Medicine.* 57 (10) October 2000: 649–655.

60 Medic, G., et al. "Short-and Long-Term Health Consequences of Sleep Disruption," *Nature and Science of Sleep.* (9) May 2017: 151–161.

61 Kahn, A., et al. "Sleep Problems in Healthy Preadolescents," *Pediatrics.* 84 (3) September 1989: 542–546. pubmed.ncbi.nlm.nih.gov/2788868/.

62 Eugene, A. R. and Masiak, J. "The Neuroprotective Aspects of Sleep," *MEDtube Science.* 3 (1) March 2015: 35–40. ncbi.nlm.nih.gov/pmc/articles/PMC4651462/.

63 Diekelmann, S. "Sleep for Cognitive Enhancement," *Frontiers in Systems Neuroscience.* 8, April 2014.

64 Wennberg, A. M. V., et al. "Sleep Disturbance, Cognitive Decline, and Dementia: A Review," *Seminars in Neurology.* 37 (4) August 2017: 395–406.

65 Loddo, G. et al. "The Treatment of Sleep Disorders in Parkinson's Disease: From Research to Clinical Practice," *Frontiers in Neurology.* 8, February 2017: 1664–2295.

66 Guarnieri, B. and Sorbi, S. "Sleep and Cognitive Decline: A Strong Bidirectional Relationship. It Is Time for Specific Recommendations on Routine Assessment and the Management of Sleep Disorders in Patients with Mild Cognitive Impairment and Dementia." *European Neurology*. 2015, 74-43-48, karger.com/Article/FullText/434629.

67 Roth, T. "Insomnia: Definition, Prevalence, Etiology, and Consequences." Published November 14, 2019. pubmed.ncbi.nlm.nih.gov/17824495/.

68 Roth, T. "Insomnia: Definition, Prevalence, Etiology, and Consequences." *Journal of Clinical Sleep Medicine.* Published online: November 14, 2019. jcsm.aasm.org/doi/10.5664/jcsm.26929

69 . Fortier-Brochu, E. and Morin, C. M. "Cognitive Impairment in Individuals with Insomnia: Clinical Significance and Correlates," *Sleep*. 37 (11) November 2014: 1787–1798.

70 Olaithe, M. et al. "Cognitive Dysfunction in Insomnia Phenotypes: Further Evidence for Different Disorders," *Frontiers in Psychiatry.* 12, July 2021.

71 Kawano, T., et al. "ER Proteostasis Regulators Cell-non-autonomously Control Sleep." *Cell Rep*. 42 (3) 2023:112267.

72 Nadeem, R. et al. "Serum Inflammatory Markers in Obstructive Sleep Apnea: A Meta-Analysis." *Journal of Clinical Sleep Medicine*. 9 (10): 1003–1012.

73 "Highlighting the Importance of Healthy Sleep Patterns in the Risk of Adult Asthma" *BMJ.* Open Respir Res 2023.

74 Oyetakin-White, P., et al. "Does Poor Sleep Quality Affect Skin Ageing?" *Clinical and Experimental Dermatology.* 40 (1) January 2015: 17–22.

75 "Association of Severe Sleep Apnea and Elevated Blood Pressure Despite Anti-hypertensives Medication Use." *JCSM*. 10 (8) 2014.
76 "Prospective Study of the Association of Sleep Apnea and Hypertension" *NEJM*. 200 (342): 1378–1384.
77 "What Happens When You Sleep?" Sleep Foundation. Updated August 29, 2022. sleepfoundation.org/how-sleep-works/what-happens-when-you-sleep.

Chapter 5: Sleep and Mental Health

78 Brabant, G., et al. "Physiologic Regulation of Circadian and Pulsatile Thyrotropin Secretion in Normal Man and Woman." *The Journal of Clinical Endocrinology & Metabolism*. February 1, 1990. 70 (2): 403–409.
79 Cleveland Clinic. "Sleep Anxiety." my.clevelandclinic.org/health/diseases/21543-sleep-anxiety.
80 Cleveland Clinic. "What Is Stress?" my.clevelandclinic.org/health/articles/11874-stress
81 National Institute of Mental Health. "What Is Anxiety?" nimh.nih.gov/health/topics/anxiety-disorders
82 "Anxiety Disorders," National Alliance on Mental Illness, nami.org/About-Mental-Illness/Mental-Health-Conditions/Anxiety-Disorders.
83 National Institute of Mental Health. "Any Anxiety Disorder: Definitions." nimh.nih.gov/health/statistics/any-anxiety-disorder.
84 Ibid.
85 Suni, E. "Anxiety and Sleep." Sleep Foundation. sleepfoundation.org/mental-health/anxiety-and-sleep.
86 *UN News* (United Nations). "Some 300-Million People Suffer from Depression, UN Warns Ahead of World Health Day." March 31, 2017. news.un.org/en/story/2017/03/554462.
87 *ABC News*. "Almost 7 in 10 Adults Dissatisfied with Their Sleep Experience Mild Depression: Poll." March 17, 2023. abcnews.go.com/Health/video/7-10-adults-dissatisfied-sleep-experience-mild-depression-97940606.
88 Krouse, L. "The Link Between Sleep and Depression," Very Well Health. Updated February 7, 2021. verywellhealth.com/depression-and-sleep-5093051.

Chapter 6: Sleep, Weight Gain, and Weight Loss

89 Centers for Disease Control and Prevention. "Adult Obesity Facts." Last updated May 17, 2022. cdc.gov/obesity/data/adult.html

90 Crispim, C. A., et al. "Relationship Between Food Intake and Sleep Pattern in Healthy Individuals." *Journal of Clinical Sleep Medicine.* 7 (6) December 2011: 659–664.

91 O'Connor, A. "How Foods May Affect Our Sleep." *New York Times*, January 1, 2021. nytimes.com/2020/12/10/well/eat/sleep-foods-diet.html.

92 Serta. "Does Sugar Keep You Awake?" Published December 2, 2022. serta.com.ph/does-sugar-keep-you-awake/.

93 Sejbuk, M. "Sleep Quality: A Narrative Review on Nutrition, Stimulants, and Physical Activity as Important Factors." *Nutrients.* 14 (9) May 2022: 1912.

94 El Mlili, N., et al. "Hair Cortisol Concentration as a Biomarker of Sleep Quality and Related Disorders." *Life (Basel).* 11 (2) January 2021: 81.

95 Stierman, B., et al. "National Health and Nutrition Examination Survey 2017–March 2020 Prepandemic Data Files Development of Files and Prevalence Estimates for Selected Health Outcomes." June 14, 2021. pubmed.ncbi.nlm.nih.gov/35593699/.

96 Sekine, M., et al. "A Dose-Response Relationship Between Short Sleeping Hours and Childhood Obesity: Results of the Toyama Birth Cohort Study," *Child: Care, Health and Development.* 28 (2) March 2002: 163–170.

97 Robards, K. "Late Bedtimes Linked with Childhood Obesity." American Academy of Sleep Medicine. Published February 5, 2021. sleepeducation.org/late-bedtimes-linked-childhood-obesity/.

98 Xiu, L., et al. "Sleep and Adiposity in Children From 2 to 6 Years of Age," *Pediatrics.* 145 (3) March 2020. pubmed.ncbi.nlm.nih.gov/32071262/.

99 Crispim, C. A., et al. "Relationship Between Food Intake and Sleep Pattern in Healthy Individuals." *Journal of Clinical Sleep Medicine.* 07 (06) December 2011: 659–664.

100 Do Vale Cardoso Lopes, T., et al. "Eating Late Negatively Affects Sleep Pattern and Apnea Severity in Individuals with Sleep Apnea." *Journal of Clinical Sleep Medicine.* 15, no. 03, March 2019: 383–392.

101 ScienceDirect. "Heartburn." sciencedirect.com/topics/medicine-and-dentistry/heartburn.

102 Mayo Clinic. "Gastroesophageal Reflux Disease (GERD)." Published January 4, 2023. mayoclinic.org/diseases-conditions/gerd/symptoms-causes/syc-20361940.

103 Gurges, P., et al. "Relationship Between Gastroesophageal Reflux Disease and Objective Sleep Quality." *Journal of Clinical Sleep Medicine.* 18 (12) December 2022: 2731–2738.

104 Fry, A. "Obesity and Sleep," Sleep Foundation. Last updated April 18, 2022. sleepfoundation.org/physical-health/obesity-and-sleep.

Chapter 7: Sleep and Sexual Health

105 National Sleep Foundation. "The Link between Nutrition and Sleep." Published November 12, 2020. thensf.org/the-link-between-nutrition-and-sleep/.

106 Suni, E. "The Relationship Between Sex and Sleep." Sleep Foundation. Last modified February 8, 2023. sleepfoundation.org/physical-health/sex-sleep.

107 National Institute of Diabetes and Digestive and Kidney Diseases. "Symptoms & Causes of Erectile Dysfunction." niddk.nih.gov/health-information/urologic-diseases/erectile-dysfunction/symptoms-causes.

108 Yetman, D. "Is Erectile Dysfunction Common? Stats, Causes, and Treatment." Healthline. Published March 5, 2020. healthline.com/health/how-common-is-ed.

109 Baldwin, K., et al. "Under-Reporting of Erectile Dysfunction Among Men with Unrelated Urologic Conditions." *International Journal of Impotence Research.* 15 (2) April 2003: 87–89.

110 Elterman, D. S., et al. "The Quality of Life and Economic Burden of Erectile Dysfunction," *Research and Reports in Urology.* 13, February 2021: 79–86.

111 Wagner G., et al. "Impact of Erectile Dysfunction on Quality of Life: Patient and Partner Perspectives." *International Journal of Impotence Research.* 2000:12 (Suppl 4). S144–S146.

112 Reishtein, J. L., et al. "Outcome of CPAP Treatment on Intimate and Sexual Relationships in Men with Obstructive Sleep Apnea," *Journal of Clinical Sleep Medicine.* 06 (03) June 2010: 221–226.

113 Hirshkowitz, M., et al. "Prevalence of Sleep Apnea in Men with Erectile Dysfunction." *Urology.* 36 (3) September 1990: 232–234.

114 Boué, S. M., et al. "Estrogenic and Antiestrogenic Activities of Phytoalexins from Red Kidney Bean (*Phaseolus vulgaris* L.)." *Journal of Agricultural and Food Chemistry.* 59 (1) December 2010: 112–120.

115 Kalmbach, D. A. "Sleep on Female Sexual Response and Behavior: A Pilot Study." *Wiley Online Library.* 12 (5) March 2015: 1221–1232.

116 Kling, J. M., et al. "Associations of Sleep and Female Sexual Function: Good Sleep Quality Matters." *Menopause.* 28 (6) June 2021: 619–625.

117 Subramanian, S., et al. "Sexual Dysfunction in Women with Obstructive Sleep Apnea." *Sleep and Breathing.* 14, 2010: 59–62.

118 Chen, Q., et.al. "Inverse U-shaped Association between Sleep Duration and Semen Quality: Longitudinal Observational Study (MARHCS) in Chongqing, China." *Sleep.* 39 (1) January 2016: 79–86.

119 Kloss, J. D., et al. "Sleep, Sleep Disturbance and Fertility in Women." *Sleep Medicine Reviews.* 22, October 2014: 78–87.

120 Zhou, X., et al. "Association of Obstructive Sleep Apnea Risk with Depression and Anxiety Symptoms in Women with Polycystic Ovary Syndrome," *Journal of Clinical Sleep Medicine.* 17 (10) October 2021: 2041–2047.

121 Lin, L., et al. "Somatic Symptoms, Psychological Distress and Sleep Disturbance among Infertile Women with Intrauterine Insemination Treatment." *Journal of Clinical Nursing.* 23 (11-12) July 2013: 1677–1684.

122 American Academy of Sleep Medicine. "Men Using CPAP See Improvement in Sexual Function, Satisfaction." Published June 13, 2012. aasm.org/men-using-cpap-see-improvement-in-sexual-function-satisfaction/.

123 Jara, S. M. et al. "Association of Continuous Positive Airway Pressure Treatment with Sexual Quality of Life in Patients with Sleep Apnea: Follow-Up Study of a Randomized Clinical Trial." *JAMA Otolaryngology, Head & Neck Surgery.* 144 (7) July 2018: 587–593.

124 Grech, A., et al. "Adverse Effects of Testosterone Replacement Therapy: An Update on the Evidence and Controversy." *Therapeutic Advances in Drug Safety.* 5 (5) 2014: 190–200.

125 Parish, J. M. "The Pursuit of Happiness: Sleep Apnea, Sex and Sleepiness." *Journal of Clinical Sleep Medicine.* Vol, 6, No.3, 2010.

Chapter 8: Sleep and Children

126 Centers for Disease Control and Prevention. "Are You Getting Enough Sleep?" cdc.gov/sleep/features/getting-enough-sleep.html.

127 Pacheco, D. "Children and Sleep." Sleep Foundation. sleepfoundation.org/children-and-sleep.

128 Owens, J. A., et al. "Evaluation and Treatment of Children and Adolescents With Excessive Daytime Sleepiness," *Sage Journals, Clinical Pediatrics.* 59 (4-5) March 13, 2020.

129 Goel, A. "Reasons for a Monthly Visit to a Pediatrician," lybrate.com/topic/reasons-for-a-monthly-visit-to-a-pediatrician/020673c9aa21cfb9f8ca85178cff3abb.

130 Autism Speaks. "Sleep." autismspeaks.org/sleep.

131 O'Brien, L. M. "The Neurocognitive Effects of Sleep Disruption in Children and Adolescents." *Child and Adolescent Psychiatric Clinics of North America.* 18 (4) October 2009: 813–823.

132 National Institutes of Health. "Kids' Sleep Linked to Brain Health." newsinhealth.nih.gov/2022/10/kids-sleep-linked-brain-health

133 McGreevey, S. "Study Flags Later Risks for Sleep-Deprived Kids." *The Harvard Gazette.* Published March 10, 2017. news.harvard.edu/gazette/story/2017/03/study-flags-later-risks-for-sleep-deprived-kids/.

134 Contie, V. "Children's Sleep Linked to Brain Development." National Institutes of Health. Published August 30, 2022. nih.gov/news-events/nih-research-matters/children-s-sleep-linked-brain-development.

135 Cleveland Clinic. "Restless Legs Syndrome (RLS) in Children and Adolescents." my.clevelandclinic.org/health/diseases/14309-restless-legs-syndrome-rls-in-children-and-adolescents.

136 Restless Legs Syndrome Foundation, Inc. "Frequently Asked Questions." rls.org/understanding-rls/faq.

137 National Institute of Neurological Disorders and Stroke. "Restless Legs Syndrome." ninds.nih.gov/health-information/disorders/restless-legs-syndrome.

138 Sleep Review. "Race is Strong Predictor for RLS." Published November 11, 2009. sleepreviewmag.com/sleep-disorders/movement-disorders/restless-legs-syndrome/race-is-strong-predictor-for-rls/.

139 Koo, B. B. "Restless Legs Syndrome: Relationship Between Prevalence and Latitude." *Sleep & Breathing, Schlaf & Atmung.* 16 (4) 2012: 1237–1245.

140 Krzysztof, K., et al. "Cognitive Deficits in Adults with Obstructive Sleep Apnea Compared to Children and Adolescents." *Journal of Neural Transmission.* 124 (1) February 2017: 187–201.

141 Kheirandish-Gozal, L., et al. "Preliminary Functional MRI Neural Correlates of Executive Functioning and Empathy in Children with Obstructive Sleep Apnea." *Sleep.* 37, March 2014: 587–592.

142 Perez-Lloret, S., et al. "A Multi-Step Pathway Connecting Short Sleep Duration to Daytime Somnolence, Reduced Attention, and Poor Academic Performance: An Exploratory Cross-Sectional Study in Teenagers." *Journal of Clinical Sleep Medicine.* 09 (05) May 2013: 469–473.

143 Wheaton, A. G. and Claussen, A. H. "Short Sleep Duration Among Infants, Children, and Adolescents Aged 4 Months-17 Years—United States, 2016–2018." *Morbidity and Mortality Weekly Report.* 70 (38) September 2021: 1315–1321.

144 Centers for Disease Control and Prevention. "How Much Sleep Do I Need?" cdc.gov/sleep/about_sleep/how_much_sleep.html.

145 Wheaton, A. G. and Claussen, A. H. "Short Sleep Duration Among Infants, Children, and Adolescents Aged 4 Months-17 Years—United States, 2016-2018." *Morbidity and Mortality Weekly Report.* 70 (38) September 2021: 1315–1321.

146 Gradisar, M., et al. "Recent Worldwide Sleep Patterns and Problems during Adolescence: A Review and Meta-Analysis of Age, Region, and Sleep." *Sleep Med.* 12, 2021:110–118.

147 Payton, L. T. "Your Kid is Losing the Equivalent of One Night's Sleep Every Week Because They Are Glued to Their Phones, New Study Reveals." *Fortune.* Published September 19, 2022. fortune.com/well/2022/09/19/kid-losing-sleep-social-media/.

148 Moyer, M. W. "Kids as Young as 8 Are Using Social Media More Than Ever, Study Finds." *New York Times,* March 24, 2022. nytimes.com/2022/03/24/well/family/child-social-media-use.html.

149 McCarthy, C. "New Advice on Melatonin Use in Children." *Harvard Health.* October 6, 2022. health.harvard.edu/blog/new-advice-on-melatonin-use-in-children-202210062832.

150 Ibid.

Chapter 9: Sleep and Teens

151 American Academy of Child and Adolescent Psychiatry. "Screen Time and Children." aacap.org/AACAP/Families_and_Youth/Facts_for_Families/FFF-Guide/Children-And-Watching-TV-054.aspx.

152 Meadows, A. "Delayed Sleep-Wake Phase Syndrome." Sleep Foundation. sleepfoundation.org/delayed-sleep-wake-phase-syndrome.

153 Onion, A. "Are You a Night Owl? It May Be a Gene Mutation." *Live Science*. Published April 6, 2017. livescience.com/58573-delayed-sleep-phase-disorder-linked-to-gene-mutation.html.

154 Gradisar, M., et al. "Recent Worldwide Sleep Patterns and Problems During Adolescence: A Review and Meta-Analysis of Age, Region, and Sleep." *Sleep Medicine*. 12 (2) February 2011: 110–118.

155 Moore, M. and Meltzer, L. J. "The Sleepy Adolescent: Causes and Consequences of Sleepiness in Teens." *Paediatric Respiratory Reviews*. 9 (2) June 2008: 114–121.

156 Wolfson, A. R. and Carskadon, M. A. "Sleep Schedules and Daytime Functioning in Adolescents." *Child Development*. 69 (4) 1998: 875–887.

157 Drake, C. et al. "The Pediatric Daytime Sleepiness Scale (PDSS): Sleep Habits and School Outcomes in Middle-School Children." *Sleep*. 26 (4) January 2003: 455–458.

158 Perez-Chada, D., et al. "Sleep Disordered Breathing and Daytime Sleepiness Are Associated with Poor Academic Performance in Teenagers. A Study Using the Pediatric Daytime Sleepiness Scale (PDSS)." *Sleep*. 30, December 2007: 1698–1703.

159 Short, M. A., et al. "Sleep on Adolescent Depressed Mood, Alertness and Academic Performance." *Journal of Adolescence*. 36 (6) December 2013: 1025–1033.

160 Wolfson, A. R. and Carskadon, M. A. "Understanding Adolescent's Sleep Patterns and School Performance: A Critical Appraisal." *Sleep Medicine Reviews*. 7 (6) December 2003: 491–506.

161 Watson, N. F. et al. "Delaying Middle School and High School Start Times Promotes Student Health and Performance: An American Academy of Sleep Medicine Position Statement." pubmed.ncbi.nlm.nih.gov/28416043/.

Chapter 10: Sleep and Women

162 Lo, S. H., et.al. "Gender Differences in Adolescent Sleep Disturbance and Treatment Response to Smartphone App–Delivered Cognitive Behavioral Therapy for Insomnia: Exploratory Study." *JMIR Formative Research*. March 23, 2021. ncbi.nlm.nih.gov/pmc/articles/PMC8075040/.

163 Zeng, L., et.al. "Gender Difference in the Prevalence of Insomnia: A Meta-Analysis of Observational Studies." *Frontiers in Psychiatry*, November 20, 2020, ncbi.nlm.nih.gov/pmc/articles/PMC7714764/.

164 Howard M. Kravitz and Joffe, H. "Sleep During the Perimenopause: A SWAN Story." *Obstetrics and Gynecology Clinics of North America*. 38 (3) September 2011: 567–586.

165 Sunset Sleep Diagnostics. "Sleep in Women." March 14, 2014. sunsetsleepdiagnostics.com/features/sleep-in-women.

166 Nowakowski, S., et.al. "Sleep and Women's Health." Sleep Medicine Research, June 30, 2013. sleepmedres.org/journal/view.php

167 Jehan, S., et.al. "Sleep and Premenstrual Syndrome." *Journal of Sleep and Medicine Disorders*. August 3, 2016. ncbi.nlm.nih.gov/pmc/articles/PMC5323065/.

168 Jones, H. J., et al. "Sleep Disturbances in Midlife Women at the Cusp of the Menopausal Transition." *Journal of Clinical Sleep Medicine*. 14 (07) 2018: 1127–1133.

169 "Can My Diet Help with Sleep Apnea? Ask a Nutritionist." Barrier Islands Free Medical Clinic. January 17, 2023. bifmc.org/can-my-diet-help-with-sleep-apnea-ask-a-nutritionist/.

170 Sleep Foundation. "Night Sweats: Causes and How to Stop Them." April 6, 2023. sleepfoundation.org/night-sweats.

171 Summer, J. and DeBanto, J. "What Causes Night Sweats in Women?" Sleep Foundation. April 6, 2023. sleepfoundation.org/night-sweats/women.

172 Sleep Foundation. "Night Sweats: Causes and How to Stop Them." April 6, 2023. sleepfoundation.org/night-sweats.

173 The Family Institute at Northwestern University. "Managing the Effects of Social Media on Teen Girls." Published March 11, 2020. counseling.northwestern.edu/blog/effects-social-media-teen-girls/.

174 Won, C. H. J. "Sleeping for Two: The Great Paradox of Sleep in Pregnancy." *Journal of Clinical Sleep Medicine*. 11 (06) 2015: 593–594.

175 Ebert, R. M., et al. "Minimal Effect of Daytime Napping Behavior on Nocturnal Sleep in Pregnant Women." *Journal of Clinical Sleep Medicine*. 11 (6) 2015: 635–643.

176 Beddoe, A. E., et al. "Effects of Mindful Yoga on Sleep in Pregnant Women: A Pilot Study." *Biological Research for Nursing*. 11 (4) 2010: 363–370.

177 Lee, S. and Hsu, H. "Stress and Health-Related Well-Being Among Mothers with a Low Birth Weight Infant: The Role of Sleep," *Social Science & Medicine*. February 2, 2012. ncbi.nlm.nih.gov/pmc/articles/PMC3464912/.

178 Smith, J. P. and Forrester, R. I. "Association Between Breastfeeding and New Mothers' Sleep: A Unique Australian Time Use Study." *International Breastfeeding Journal*. January 6, 2021.

179 Richter, D., et al. "Long-term Effects of Pregnancy and Childbirth on Sleep Satisfaction and Duration of First-Time and Experienced Mothers and Fathers." *Sleep*. 42 (4) 2019.

180 Johnson, D. A., et al. "Environmental Determinants of Insufficient Sleep and Sleep Disorders: Implications for Population Health. *Current Epidemiology Reports, 5* (2) 2019: 61–69.

Chapter 11: Sleep and Older Adults

181 Sleep Health Foundation. "Advanced Sleep Phase Disorder." Last modified March 10, 2020. sleephealthfoundation.org.au/advanced-sleep-phase-disorder-aspd.html.

182 Stanford Health Care. "Advanced Sleep Phase Syndrome." stanfordhealthcare.org/medical-conditions/sleep/advanced-sleep-phase-syndrome.html.

183 Office of the Assistant Secretary for Health. "New Surgeon General Advisory Raises Alarm about the Devastating Impact of the Epidemic of Loneliness and Isolation in the United States." May 3, 2023. hhs.gov/about/news/2023/05/03/new-surgeon-general-advisory-raises-alarm-about-devastating-impact-epidemic-loneliness-isolation-united-states.html.

184 Kline, L. R. "Clinical Presentation and Diagnosis of Obstructive Sleep Apnea in Adults." UpToDate. Last modified January 13, 2023. uptodate.com/contents/clinical-presentation-and-diagnosis-of-obstructive-sleep-apnea-in-adults.

185 Nguyen, V., et al. "Insomnia in Older Adults." *Current Geriatrics Reports.* 8 (4) October 2019: 271–290.

Chapter 12: Sleep, Performance, and Work

186 Parkes, D. "Murdoc's Decision: In Retrospect." The Life and Mystery of First Officer William Murdoch. williammurdoch.net/man-07_decision_in_retrospect.html.

187 Tikkanen, A. "Titanic," *Encyclopedia Britannica.* Last modified March 3, 2023. britannica.com/topic/Titanic.

188 Wilkens, J. "The Navy Fought Sleep with Benzedrine and Strong Coffee." *The San Diego Union Tribute.* April 9, 2021. sandiegouniontribune.com/news/military/story/2021-04-09/navy-combats-sleep-deprivation

189 Varghese, C. and Shankar, U. "Passenger Vehicle Occupant Fatalities by Day and Night—A Contrast." *NHTSA.* May 2007. crashstats.nhtsa.dot.gov/api/public/viewpublication/810637.

190 Gottlieb, D. J., et al. "Sleep Deficiency and Motor Vehicle Crash Risk in the General Population: A Prospective Cohort Study." *BMC Med.* 16 (1) March 2018: 44.

191 Institute of Medicine (US) Committee on Sleep Medicine and Research. "Functional and Economic Impact of Sleep Loss and Sleep-Related Disorders." *Sleep Disorders and Sleep Deprivation: An Unmet Public Health Problem*, ed. H. R. Colten and B. M. Altevogt. ncbi.nlm.nih.gov/books/NBK19958/

192 Swanson, L. M., et al. "Sleep Disorders and Work Performance: Findings from the 2008 National Sleep Foundation Sleep in America Poll." *Journal of Sleep Research.* 20 (3) September 2011: 487–94.

193 Léger, D. et al. "Medical and Socio-Professional Impact of Insomnia." *Sleep.* 25 (6) September 2002: 625–629. pubmed.ncbi.nlm.nih.gov/12224841/.

194 Shahly, V., et al. "The Associations of Insomnia with Costly Workplace Accidents and Errors: Results from the America Insomnia Survey." *Archives of General Psychiatry.* 69 (10) October 2012: 1054–1063.

195 RAND Corporation. "Lack of Sleep Costing US Economy Up to $411 Billion per Year." ScienceDaily. Published November 30, 2016. sciencedaily.com/releases/2016/11/161130130826.htm.

196 Metlaine, A. et al. "Socioeconomic Impact of Insomnia in Working Populations." *Industrial Health.* 43 (1) March 2006: 11–19.

197 Jaslow, R. "Sleep Disorders Tally $94.9 Billion in Health Care Costs Each Year." Massey Eye and Ear. Published May 7, 2021. masseyeandear.org/news/press-releases/2021/05/sleep-disorders-tally-94-billion-in-health-care-costs-each-year

198 Alton, L. "Why Lack of Sleep Is Costing Us Billions of Dollars." *NBC News.* Published June 2, 2017. www.nbcnews.com/better/better/why-lack-sleep-costing-us-billions-dollars-ncna767571

199 Hafner, M. et al. *The Societal And Economic Burden of Insomnia in Adults: An International Study.*" Santa Monica, CA: RAND Corporation. 2023. rand.org/pubs/research_reports/RRA2166-1.html.

200 Pinholster, G. "Sleep Deprivation Described as a Serious Public Health Problem." American Association for the Advancement of Science. Last modified March 14, 2014. aaas.org/news/sleep-deprivation-described-serious-public-health-problem.

201 Centers for Disease Control and Prevention. "1 in 3 Adults Don't Get Enough Sleep." Last updated February 16, 2016. cdc.gov/media/releases/2016/p0215-enough-sleep.html.

202 Daley, M., et al. "The Economic Burden of Insomnia: Direct and Indirect Costs for Individuals with Insomnia Syndrome, Insomnia Symptoms, and Good Sleepers." *Sleep.* 32 (1) January 2009: 55–64. ncbi.nlm.nih.gov/pmc/articles/PMC2625324/.

203 Kaliyaperumal, D., et al. "Effects of Sleep Deprivation on the Cognitive Performance of Nurses Working in Shift." *Journal of Clinical and Diagnostic Research.* 11 (8) August 2017: CC01–CC03.

204 Garbarino, S., et al. "Insomnia Is Associated with Road Accidents. Further Evidence from a Study on Truck Drivers," *PloS One.* 12 (10) October 2017: e0187256.

205 Goel, N., et al. "Neurocognitive Consequences of Sleep Deprivation." *Seminars in Neurology.* 29 (4) September 2009: 320–339.

206 Hafner, M., et al. "Why Sleep Matters—The Economic Costs of Insufficient Sleep: A Cross-Country Comparative Analysis." *Rand Health Quarterly.* 6 (4) January 2017: 11. ncbi.nlm.nih.gov/pmc/articles/PMC5627640/.

207 Torborg, L. "Mayo Clinic Q&A: Neck Size One Risk Factor for Obstructive Sleep Apnea." Published June 15, 2015. newsnetwork.mayoclinic.org/discussion/mayo-clinic-q-and-a-neck-size-one-risk-factor-for-obstructive-sleep-apnea/

208 Suni, E. and Vyas, N. "How Lack of Sleep Impacts Cognitive Performance and Focus." SleepFoundation.org. sleepfoundation.org/sleep-deprivation/lack-of-sleep-and-cognitive-impairment

209 Gupta, A., et al. "Shift Work: A Perspective on Shift Work Disorder—Is Prevention the Answer?" *Journal of Clinical Sleep Medicine.* 15 (12) December 2019: 1863–1865.

210 Swinbourne, R., et al. "Prevalence of Poor Sleep Quality, Sleepiness, and Obstructive Sleep Apnoea Risk Factors in Athletes." *European Journal of Sport Science.* 16 (7). Published online December 23, 2015.

211 Fullagar, H. H., et al. "Sleep and Athletic Performance: The Effects of Sleep Loss on Exercise Performance, and Physiological and Cognitive Responses to Exercise." *Sports Medicine.* 45 (2) February 2015: 161–186.

212 Azboy, O. and Kaygisiz, Z. "Effects of sleep deprivation on cardiorespiratory functions of the runners and volleyball players during rest and exercise." *Acta Physiol Hung.* 96 (1). March 1, 2009: 29–36. pubmed.ncbi.nlm.nih.gov/19264040/

213 Halson, S.L. "Sleep in Elite Athletes and Nutritional Interventions to Enhance Sleep." *Sports Medicine*. Published online May 3, 2014. 44 (Suppl 1): 13–23.

214 Smith, R. S., et al. "Circadian Misalignment on Athletic Performance in Professional Football Players." *Sleep.* 36 (12) December 2013: 1999–2001.

215 Lee, A. and Galvez, J. C. "Jet Lag in Athletes." *Sports Health.* 4 (3) May 2012: 211–216.

216 Ibid.

217 Smith R. S., et al. "Circadian Rhythms and Enhanced Athletic Performance in the National Football League." *Sleep*. 1997 (20): 362–365.

218 Watson, A. M. "Sleep and Athletic Performance." *Current Sports Medicine Reports.* 16 (6) 2017: 413–418. pubmed.ncbi.nlm.nih.gov/29135639/

219 Charest, J. and Grandner, M. A. "Sleep and Athletic Performance: Impacts on Physical Performance, Mental Performance, Injury Risk and Recovery, and Mental Health." *Sleep Medicine Clinics*. 15 (1) March 2020: 41–57.

220 Knufinke, M., et al. "Self-Reported Sleep Quantity, Quality and Sleep Hygiene in Elite Athletes." *Journal of Sleep Research.* 27 (1): 78–85.

221 Milewski, M. et al. "Chronic Lack of Sleep Is Associated with Increased Sports Injuries in Adolescent Athletes." *Journal of Pediatric Orthopedics.* 34 (2) March 2014: 129–133.

222 Rabin, J. M., et al. "Assessment of Sleep Health in Collegiate Athletes Using the Athlete Sleep Screening Questionnaire." *Journal of Clinical Sleep Medicine.* 16 (8) August 2020: 1349–1356.

223 Minnesota Sleep Society. "Sports Related Injury and Performance." mnsleep.net/school-start-time-toolkit/why-improve-sleep-for-teenage-students/evidence-confirms-link-between-teen-sleep-biology-and-improved-outcomes/sports-related-injury-and-performance/.

224 Watson, A. M. "Sleep and Athletic Performance." *Current Sports Medicine Reports.* 16 (6) 2017: 413–418.

225 Ibid.

226 Gallagher, J. "A Daytime Nap Is Good for the Brain." *BBC News*. June 20, 2023. bbc.com/news/health-65950168.

227 Ibid.

Chapter 13: Sleep Treatments

228 VeryWell. "9 Breathing Exercises to Relieve Anxiety." Updated January 27, 2023. verywellmind.com/abdominal-breathing-2584115

229 Wilson, D. R. "How to Use 4-7-8 Breathing for Anxiety." Updated January 11, 2023. medicalnewstoday.com/articles/324417

230 American College of Physicians. "ACP Recommends Cognitive Behavioral Therapy as Initial Treatment for Chronic Insomnia." May 3, 2016. acponline.org/acp-newsroom/acp-recommends-cognitive-behavioral-therapy-as-initial-treatment-forchronic-insomnia

231 For the sake of transparency, I have given presentations on Quvivig® (daridorexant), a registered trademark of Idorsia Pharmaceuticals Ltd.

Chapter 14: Conclusion

232 Shin, J. E. and Kim, J. K. "How a Good Sleep Predicts Life Satisfaction: The Role of Zero-Sum Beliefs About Happiness." *Frontiers in Psychology.* 2018 (9): 1589. Published online 28 August 2018. ncbi.nlm.nih.gov/pmc/articles/PMC6121950/.

So, Now What?

Download Your FREE Special Report
The Good, the Bad, the Ugly... and the Beautiful

How a Continuous Positive Airway Pressure (CPAP) Machine Can Help You Sleep Better, Feel Sexier, and Live Longer

Are you or your partner tired of restless nights, daytime exhaustion, and disruptive snoring that makes life miserable… but hesitant to get (or use) a CPAP because of all the "issues"?

You're not alone! In my FREE special report, you'll learn how CPAP therapy can:

- Give you (and your partner) "the gift of bliss"—peaceful, uninterrupted sleep
- Restore your vitality, cognitive function, and memory
- Help you wake up feeling refreshed and energized
- Boost your mood and overall well-being throughout the day

You'll also discover…

- How to make nighttime CPAP preparation as simple as brushing your teeth
- How to reduce the adjustment period when first using your CPAP
- 5 ways to overcome CPAP "stigma"
- 10 top reasons why people abandon using their CPAP (a huge health risk!)
- How to prevent problems like "rainout" or "dry throat" before they begin
- How to clean your CPAP—and avoid the one *most dangerous* thing you can do when using a CPAP (besides not using it!)

- How to *enhance* intimacy with your partner by using a CPAP
- How to get your partner to actually *want* to use a CPAP every night without fail

Don't let one more sleepless night affect your health, your confidence, or your relationship. Using a CPAP could be your ticket to a sleeping better, feeling sexier, and living longer! To claim your FREE special report, visit **SleepFixAcademy.com/CPAP** or simply scan the QR code below.